Living with Peanut Anaphylaxis

or other Life Threatening Food Allergies

Michael Sporer

Printed by CreateSpace
Available on Kindle and other devices

ISBN: 1512050814
ISBN-13: 978-1512050813

Cover artwork by T. Pastoria

This book is dedicated:

> To every parent who is striving so that their child can live the life that they dream of for them.
>
> To every child who held their parents hand and told them that it will be OK.
>
> To my mother who showed me how to hold on to hope when it seems hopeless.
>
> To my father, my beacon, who leads me down the right path.
>
> To 110 of my friends who showed me everything else is pointless.
>
> *Most of all, to my Angels.*

Forward

I started blogging on March 20th, 2015. ... I wasn't planning to write a book, but a blog isn't something you can hold in your hand, write in the margins or gets marked with a coffee stain on that one day when everything seems to be going so right yet so wrong all at the same time. The book has been edited for clarity to try to help you find your path on this journey you are about to embark on.

Will you find answers? Maybe. My goal is to help you find the right questions, to give you the confidence to advocate, and *how to advocate*. You will take your own path to get there; everyone is different. What has worked for me might not work for you, regardless; we are all in this together.

What I write will no doubt attract criticism. I'm ok with that. This is my story and how I managed to survive in some unforgiving circumstances. At one point I had to decide if it was more important to be nice and diplomatic or to protect my health and well being. I chose the latter. I chose life, I chose me.

I'd like to say these skills have served me well and kept me alive, but the truth is I was surviving before I learned these skills. I may have been surviving, but I wasn't *living*. This is my story of how I made it from merely surviving all the way to **Living with Peanut Anaphylaxis**.

Table of Contents

Forward v

Introduction ix

Chapter 1 - My Back-story 1

   As a young adult...2

   The first time… 4

   My last anaphylactic reaction.............................9

Chapter 2 - Living with Peanut Anaphylaxis......... 17

   My safe bubble, my prison.....................................17

   Hope is empowering...18

   Anaphylaxis 101...19

   Allergen Exposure and Allergen Loading 25

Chapter 3 - Well meant advice 29

   Peanut is not a nut...29

   Explaining your avoidance reasoning: Sometimes it's
      just the inconvenience 30

   The inconvenience of a reaction: reality 34

   Dining out: Step 1..36

   Flying with PA: advice 39

   Becoming your own advocate 43

Chapter 4 - Surviving with Peanut Anaphylaxis .. 45

   Eating out – When outside your safe bubble.............45

   Airborne Allergy Discovery at 36,000 feet 51

   Flying with PA: Customer service hell........................53

   Bad Doggy Kisses...63

Chapter 5 - There is one question that you should NEVER ask 67

The Food Industry 68

Airlines 68

Side Effects ... and a whole lot more 72

Chapter 6 - Protecting the ones we love 75

Insulin Angel Medication Tracker 76

The Veta™ is a Smart case for remote monitoring of your child's Epi-pen..............................77

Chapter 7 - My OIT Story, the beginning.............. 79

Clinical Trial Acceptance Testing 83

I was IN! 90

Glossary: 95

Resources: 97

ADVANCED Acute management of anaphylaxis guidelines 97

Social Media: 98

Facebook Groups: 98

Non Profits:...99

False Prophets: 99

Airborne Exposure Research 100

Good Doggy Kisses......................................102

Epilogue 103

Introduction

So, you just heard the dreaded news; your child has a Life Threatening Food Allergy (LTFA) and you are wondering just where to begin. Well, prepare to be inundated with information and well intentioned advice from every angle. Ultimately, you chose to be parent and everything that it entails, including the responsibility to make informed decisions. I've raised three daughters and despite my shortcomings as a parent they've turned out to be pretty darn awesome. But it wasn't easy and I couldn't have written this book even just a few years ago.

At any point in time parents are faced with too many choices, too many options. In the end there is only one path taken, one road traveled. This is a one way road and if you ever have a moment of self doubt of why you are on this road there is only one acceptable answer.

"I MADE THE BEST DECISION THAT I COULD WITH THE INFORMATION AVAILABLE TO ME AT THE TIME."

Put this in your toolbox and reach for it often. Decide that you want to learn to make better decisions in the future and stop worrying about what almost happened. LTFA is a profound, terrifying experience, and not just for the parents. Mistakes will be made, accidents happen. Learn, live, keep moving forward. There is no alternative.

My journey started 49 years ago and back then some things were quite different, some better and some worse. My three children and my wife don't have any food allergies of any sort. I have not been through the journey that you are embarking on as a parent, but I *have* been on that journey as a child, a teenager, a college student, a different kind of parent, and finally as an adult.

What I write might seem unsympathetic, but trust me, my heart breaks every time I hear about someone's life cut short by this unforgiving and uncontrolled reaction called Anaphylaxis.

Anaphylaxis itself is more a severe symptom than it is a disease. Granted, anaphylaxis can be fatal or can be counteracted by quick attention with Epinephrine, which is as close to a miracle drug as is possible today, but when you administer Epi, you are treating a symptom of the underlying problem of Life Threatening (Food) Allergies (LTFA).

What causes LTFA? How can LTFA be treated? How can LTFA be cured? These are important questions that the health industry is just beginning to understand.

In the meantime however, you have an immediate problem with no easy answers. Every child is different in the way they respond to this medical condition. As well, every child is different to how they respond to the mental and emotional burden that comes along with it. What works for one child might not apply to another, what works when they are young probably won't work when they are older. As a parent you need to remember that it's your child, not you, that has the allergy. **Never forget that.** Your job is to keep them safe, but more importantly your job is to teach them how to be safe themselves so they can live the life that you dream they will have. Teach them to advocate when they need to, and to turn away rather than be pressured into something that may cause them harm. It takes years to teach these lessons, trust me, I know. These lessons are as important as addressing the medical condition itself.

Everyone has a theory over what has caused the epidemic rise in LTFA in roughly the last decade. While I will not discuss this in the book, I encourage you to investigate at least these two possibilities:

1) Changes in vaccination protocols; not the vaccines themselves, but the increased intensities in which they are administered into our youth. Vaccines are not bad, and are intended to strengthen our auto-immune system. It's also well accepted that allergies are an auto-immune response. You should understand the changes in vaccination protocols since 1990 before you dismiss this possible contributor.

2) Genetically Modified (GMO) crops driven by big agriculture. Corporations inherently value profit above the greater good. Food allergies are an auto-immune response to … FOOD. What are we doing to our food supply? Why are food allergies rising in industrialized nations? What is the connection to industrial food production, use of pesticides, antibiotics and GMO modified crops? I have no idea. It just seems like we are playing with fire on a national or worldwide scale.

You can find more information on these topics in the reference section at the end.

Parents Warning

I'm trying to be honest, like the impact this has had on my mental health. LTFA is more than just a medical condition and it affects quality of life in every way imaginable. The anaphylaxis is scary, but you need to be strong and present for your kids. You need to control this rather than letting it control you. Most importantly is to EMPOWER your children to control and speak up for their health and safety, including the decision to start a desensitization treatment when THEY are ready. You need to let your child lead you on the journey. They will be ready to lead sooner than you think; will you be ready to let them when they want you to?

I've gotten feedback that some of what I write about is too frightening to be shared with parents who are dealing with kids with allergies. I'd rather they read about me, the boy that lived, than the **alternative**. My story will **hopefully have a happy ending** someday.

Chapter 1 - My Back-story

I want to free myself from the curse of an anaphylactic food allergy

"Did social media like Facebook and Twitter cause the revolution? No. But these tools did speed up the process by helping to organize the revolutionaries, transmit their message to the world and galvanize international support." – Wired Magazine – 2011

For quite some time thought I was either alone with this problem, or was in fact the oldest person with it. I realize now this is not the case, but when I was a kid, peanut or food allergies were not as prevalent as they are now. And there were no advocacy groups or social media to connect people together. I've heard about the 'cure' for peanut allergy for several years now, and since learning more about it in the last six months I've decided it is less risky at this point in my life to go through Immunotherapy (IT) desensitization rather than continue peanut avoidance.

I am peanut and tree nut allergic, and as far as I know have been all my life. I was raised in a meat and potatoes family, the only peanuts in the house was peanut butter for PBJ's and tree nuts were considered expensive treats only for adult consumption.

Back then processed foods may have had lower risk of cross contamination. I can't be certain, but I'd guess advances in the food industry over my lifetime probably increased the chance of cross contamination before it was recognized as a problem, and now it seems the awareness and risk has come down in the last 20 years.

I survived simply by avoidance. I used to say I didn't like the smell of peanuts and was labeled a picky eater. Now, as an adult, I can say the smell of peanuts causes me to have a sinus reaction that happens before I can actually smell the peanuts. Imagine this, **it feels like a pair of red hot six inch long needles being jammed up my nose.** But as a kid I didn't have the language to describe it, so it was just "I don't like the smell", and I would hold my nose.

My brothers and sisters would make PBJ for lunch and if the PB jar was open I'd ask them to close it. Of course, I never ate jelly either, because the PB knife went in the PB first, then the jelly, so the jelly was always contaminated. I'd eat jelly on two occasions; first, if there was a brand new jar, and second, at a restaurant with individual jelly packets.

If I ate a tree nut or anything remotely contaminated I would vomit, quite violently. Never had any reaction requiring any medical intervention, no one knew that the vomiting was an anaphylactic symptom.

This is what I remember from my childhood home.

As a young adult

In 1977, when I was twelve years old we moved out of the inner city of Detroit to a suburb. The old neighborhood was ethnically Polish and German. The only thing I couldn't or wouldn't eat was

Baklava, but besides that the menu was pretty safe. The new neighborhood had different ethnic restaurants; Asian, Mexican, Greek to name a few. I had never eaten at an Asian restaurant before and it didn't work out too well. The first time I didn't order any dish with nuts, but ended up with a very swollen face. After a while it passed and later was attributed to MSG, since that wasn't used at home. The second time at a Chinese restaurant I became nauseous on the car ride home and vomited. And that was the last time I ate Asian food for many years.

There was nothing out of the ordinary with respect to my food allergies. I had a strong avoidance ability and I just kept my food choices pretty narrow. I was never adventurous when it came to eating and I came to discover that I could detect allergens with my sinus. It wasn't the odor; rather I could detect allergic inflammation simply by airborne exposure. I recall when I was a teenager that I had gotten into the habit of smelling my food when not eating at home and was told that my behavior was rude. This was at either a friend's house at dinner or at a restaurant. Apparently sticking your face into a plate and taking a big whiff didn't pass muster, so I figured out how to be more discrete about it.

Then I went away to college, lived in a dorm. Somewhere along the way I lost the automatic vomiting reflex, I seem to think that happened in conjunction with excessive alcohol intake, either that or I just grew out of it. I never knew there was version of captain crunch with peanut flavored bits, but I found out. I got pretty good at discretely spitting food that I didn't 'like' into a napkin.

I moved into a housing cooperative and during the orientation meeting the kitchen steward asked if anyone had any food restrictions or allergies. Imagine that! People could be actually allergic to food! I had never even heard of such a thing before. This was my chance. I told the steward that I was allergic to nuts, and I was asked what happens when I eat them... "Uh, uh, jeez, I don't really know since I don't eat them." I didn't realize that vomiting was an allergic reaction, so I didn't mention that, but the attempt to describe any symptoms was met with a puzzled look. Regardless, I managed to avoid nuts for the most part until my Junior year ... until the night before spring break...

The first time...

I was getting ready for spring break my junior year and I still had a project to turn in before I could leave. I left the house after breakfast and headed up to the engineering campus, about 4 miles away by bus. I went to class and went to library/labs as needed to work on the project, skipping lunch. The coop where I lived provided room and board so I was not accustomed to buying meals. I was living on a student budget. Around dinner I was still at it, skipped dinner and finally realized I had to make the last bus back to main campus, so finished or not, I wrapped up what I was working on, turned it in and headed down to the bus stop. It was late, snowing, I was hungry, and I had to get up early tomorrow to get to the airport. I got home and the house was nearly empty, most of my housemates had left or were sleeping. There was a grad student, Mark, who was not going away for spring break. I went down to the kitchen for some food. I was famished.

When I got to the kitchen I was struck by a powerful smell. Someone had burned something... badly. Cookies ... someone had baked cookies, and they were sitting on a cookie sheet in the middle of the kitchen. Hmmm, I thought, Appetizer! So I scraped a cookie off the pan and I bit it. I swear it was 60% charcoal and 40% cookie, but I wolfed it down anyway, and I might have eaten a second, not sure, there was a horrible taste in my mouth, so I got some milk, then picked up another cookie and started scraping off the charcoal. Uh oh! ... **Peanut butter cookies.** Hmmm... and I had no idea how severe the reaction would be. My throat started itching and my first thought was to vomit, but nothing would come up, so I ate some fruit salad and tried to vomit again, nothing. Then I started to feel hot and chilled, my skin started to crawl and hives broke out on my hands. But the thing that I remember clearest was the feeling that **something terrible was happening**.

I found Mark and told him I needed to go to the hospital. He saw the look on my face and never questioned why. We got in a pickup truck and pulled out in the street. It was about 2 hilly miles to the hospital and there was 8 inches of fresh snow on the road. The streets had not been plowed. Later, Mark told me he was worried about what he would do if the truck slid off the road and got stuck in the snow. [This was about five years before the 1st hand held cell phone was even invented.] About halfway to the hospital I started feeling funny, so I told Mark everything that I knew about the situation (which wasn't much), told him my symptoms and that he had to walk me into the ER. We soon arrived and I got up to the desk and the nurse asked what was wrong. I tried to speak, but I couldn't, my throat was swelling and I couldn't vocalize. I raised my hands to my throat as if I was choking myself and Mark realized that he was my only hope. Quickly they whisked me into the ER.

ER Treatment

To the best of my knowledge I never lost consciousness. I was lying on an ER bed and medical personnel were swarming around me. They put IV's in both my arms and took my blood pressure over top of a heavy flannel shirt... I kid you not, I heard "it's forty over zero" and I thought, "That's not possible". By now I could tell I was starting to swell all over my body and a heavy weight started pushing down on my chest making it harder to breath. It wasn't that my throat was closed; rather I was starting into respiratory collapse as my lungs were filling up with fluid. While this was happening the docs and nurses weren't just standing there, it was pandemonium and here comes the medication injected into the IV which were both running wide open. First one dose in each arm, then one more (one arm) and finally I started to feel like I wasn't going to implode and I could **breathe** again.

After the first two liters of saline were gone they hooked up 2 more. Prednisone goes into the IV bag, and I start to relax. The doc checks on me and things start to settle down. I'm feeling a little tired, but I don't fall asleep.

In less than a half hour I go from feeling fine to panic in an instant, the epi had worn off and the reaction was coming back. Fortunately the nurse is right there and the doc gives me some more IV meds and I start to feel better again. Then I'm on observation for the next couple of hours. Finally they say I can leave, but first I have to get rid of 4 liters of saline which takes quite some time, so long in fact the nurse knocked on the bathroom door to make sure I was ok. I was given a prescription for prednisone and get it filled at the pharmacy.

As I was discharged they tell me to avoid eating peanuts and to see my allergist. What allergist?? I don't have an allergist. I have a couple hours before the shuttle to the airport will pick me up. So I walk out into the ER waiting room and Mark is there, waiting for me. [Mark Hall, I can never thank you enough for being there that night. Someday I hope we can meet again.] The flight to CA was uneventful. Back then the stewardess would take your drink order, and hand you the drink, a napkin and a bag of peanuts. They basically pushed peanuts into everyone's hands, even those people that wouldn't ask for them if given the choice. **No,** I really don't mind if you eat peanuts in my presence, **PROVIDED THAT YOU DON'T EXHALE.**

Was that just a bad dream?

When I returned to school I went to see the allergist and had a round of skin tests. Back then they would apply the liquid, and then come back later with a tool and scratch each site. Not very repeatable compared to what they do today. As they applied the allergens to my back one of them felt like I was being stabbed by a needle, and that was before the scratch. After time was up they started assessing the results on the 5 point scale. Some mild allergies to common airborne and seasonal things, scoring 1 to 3, but the tree nuts were 5/5. Then I watched the nurse mark off the peanut line item. She crossed out the 5 point scale and drew a wheal that was about the size of a quarter.

The consult with the allergist was pretty low key. I shouldn't eat nuts, peanuts could kill me, if I do eat them I need to seek emergency treatment right away, and here is a prescription for an Ana-kit. He even showed me how to use it. It looked pretty simple. OK, ok, fine. But that was just a fluke, I made it 20 years without a reaction, I should be able to make it 20 more. Or so I thought. One thing I did do was I always carried the Ana-kit which was a simple syringe of epinephrine, not an auto-injector and a couple tablets of anti-histamine. I decided I would not eat unless I had my Ana-kit with me. Going all day without eating makes you remember to bring it along. In the last 30 years I probably went out without it once or possibly twice.

**Food is necessary for life,
but sometimes it can kill you too.**

Management of Anaphylaxis Guidelines

I was looking for something that remotely describes my ER experience with anaphylaxis and I had to go to Australia to find it. No doubt the US legal system prevents posting information like this lest someone is then liable. Please refer to the Resources Section.

My last anaphylactic reaction

I'm not going to bore you with the details of the other reactions, just the last one I had. Well, actually I'm kidding. I've only had two reactions in my life, the first and the last, and if you read about this one you'll understand why.

Other than carrying the Ana-kit, I really didn't change much in the way that I managed my food. I was still in college and once again working late, but this time I went to a different, closer coop on campus for dinner. My house was sponsoring an open party that night, and I had the alcohol in my car, so I was going to eat, finish the project and get home. The party theme was "The (annual) **End of the World** Party". Oh, the *irony*.

The food was great and the dessert was a chocolate chip cookie in a pan. I love dark chocolate, but milk chocolate not so much. Some milk chocolate gave me a 'funny' feeling, that feeling of "you shouldn't be eating this". Was it cross contaminated? No idea, but I never had a problem with dark chocolate chips. I just thought the flavor of chocolate was inherently nutty, but I never had a problem with it. So I ate some cookie, sweet, chocolaty ...but uh oh, I got that feeling ... **"you shouldn't be eating this."**

This cookie was big enough to serve about 100 people (It was a big house.), it was over four large cookie sheets. I was talking to the president of the house and the cook. The cook said that they added a secret ingredient to the cookie dough. It was a couple tablespoons of peanut butter. I turned to the president of the house, thinking to myself, "I know how to handle this", and said I needed to go to the hospital right away. Luckily, I had a car, but I needed him to drive me. We got to the ER and remembering what had happened to Mark the previous time I told him he didn't need to wait around, but if he would please deliver the alcohol to the party for me.

I went up to the admitting desk and told the nurse what was going on.

"I am deathly allergic to peanuts and inadvertently ate some and I needed to be admitted right away."

She looked at me and handed me a clipboard with a form to fill out... **"WHAT??"** I thought.

"This is serious; I need to be admitted right away."

She asked me what my symptoms were so I told her, and she politely asked me to please fill out the form.

It was a short form and I did quickly, and they put me in a wheel chair, brought me in and placed me on a bed... **for observation**.

"Excuse me doctor, this is very serious, aren't you going to treat me?"

"I'm sorry" was the reply, "there's nothing we can do until you start showing symptoms."

So, before I continue let me say that that statement is WRONG. There is something that can be done and **ABSOLUTELY SHOULD BE DONE!**

If someone is either showing <u>anaphylactic</u> symptoms or has a prior history with a known ingestion, they should be administered using an auto-injector *IntraMuscular* Epinephrine (IM epi) as SOON AS POSSIBLE. If the victim doesn't have the medication on them then ASK EVERYONE. Most likely someone will have one. DON'T WAIT. Administer it in the *outer thigh*, <u>through the clothing</u>, hold in place for 10 seconds, Call 911 and then massage the injection site. With any medication there are risks, but administering <u>one dose</u> and then determining the next course of action is lower risk than not giving the medication. Once the medication is in the system you've bought yourself some time.

Excuse Me!

Wait a minute, the last time I was here I had all the attention in the world, this time the nurse came by every few minutes to check in on me. What don't these people understand about Emergency Room?

I wouldn't be here if it wasn't an EMERGENCY.

I was dumbfounded and confused (another anaphylaxis symptom), but frankly the reaction was progressing much slower than the previous episode. Perhaps this time wouldn't be so bad after all. I'm sitting there 10, 15, 20, 25 minutes and all I had was an itchy throat. I actually had a bunch of other real symptoms, but I just thought I was feeling them because I was scared. I didn't realize they were real symptoms.

The nurse had just checked on me again. Taken my vitals and noted in the chart. So I lay back in bed, wondering what to do next. I didn't have to wait long...

It was like I was lying on the beach, uncomfortably baking under the hot sun, when suddenly, like a tsunami, I feel this wave wash over me. I still have no explanation of what was happening, but it quickly engulfing me and it was frightening. I was feeling scared and alone, very alone, **and I needed someone, anyone to be with me.** So I sat up and bed and called out to the first person walking by "Excuse me".

I suppose it's fortunate that I did, otherwise I probably wouldn't be here today.

It was a different nurse, she turned and looked at me and cried out something, I'm not sure what, but instantly I was surrounded by medical personnel. They laid me back on the bed then flattened the bed out. It felt like they were doing the same drill as last time; dual IVs, IV epi, but to me it felt different. Very, very different. This time ...

I WAS SURE I WAS GOING TO DIE.

I didn't come to this conclusion while I was waiting. It came to me after they laid me down on the table because it felt so different than before. The speed at which the reaction came on was terrifying and it felt stronger, and felt like the ER personnel weren't going to be able to treat me fast enough to pull me back.

Did I lose consciousness? I don't think so.
Did I close my eyes and see a light? No.
Did I see an angel or God? No.
None of those. I was just certain I was going to die.

Not too long ago I was using a razor knife in my workshop trimming a piece of wood. As the knife came around the corner of the piece it was aiming at my left hand and I said to myself "I need to move my left hand", but before I could the knife slipped and in that moment of time before the knife slashed into my thumb I thought "**You idiot, you weren't careful enough, and now look what is going to happen.**"

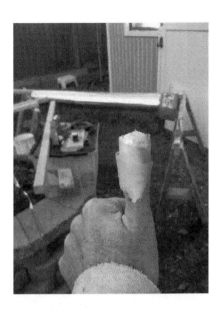

When I was lying in the ER bed that's what I thought, I wasn't careful enough, **this was all my fault** and I was going to die.

I have no idea what drowning feels like, but maybe that's what I was feeling. I was at one of the best University medical centers in the nation, miles from the nearest body of water and I was going to drown. But finally I was at peace, because at least now I wasn't alone. Someone actually cared enough to *try* to save me.

That is what the worst, scariest, loneliest feeling in the world was. Feeling like something was terribly wrong, and no one believed you, no one even cared.

The Boy Who Lived

I felt like I was skydiving naked, being chased by the medical team who was trying to catch me and get me into a parachute as we were falling through the air. They succeeded and pulled the ripcord. How close was it? I don't really know. My face was swollen and I couldn't open my eyes, so I couldn't see the ground rushing at me ... but the parachute opened and I could **breathe** again.

What was happening to me? What just happened? What's going to happen next? I tried to rest, but I couldn't.

The boomerang. What about the boomerang? You know, when the epi wears off like it did last time? Will this boomerang be the same as what happened before, or will it also be worse this around? BAM! The boomerang hit me hard, and the medical team responded.

Was it worse? I couldn't tell, I didn't care, just make it go away ... just **don't let me die ...** Why is this happening to ME??

I was exhausted. I didn't know what to do, what to think. I just needed to rest. "But there is no rest for you, my pretty", said the boomerang. This time I duck and it was a glancing blow. Me and my new friends Epi and Pred pushed the boomerang away one last time. Finally, I could rest.

MEANWHILE, BACK AT THE END OF THE WORLD PARTY:

"WHERE'S MICHAEL?" SHE ASKED MY ROOMMATE, HAVING JUST ARRIVED.

"HE'S IN THE HOSPITAL" WAS THE SLURRED REPLY.

"WHAT HAPPENED? WHY AREN'T YOU THERE WITH HIM??"

"I HAD TO BE HERE, SO I COULD TELL YOU WHERE HE WAS."

She was energetic, passionate and full of life, everything that I needed*.

When she arrived at the ER they told her she couldn't go in because she wasn't related. The nurse tried to stop her. Security tried to stop her. Everyone said 'you can't go in there'. But I was not at all surprised when I saw her face, my angel. "What took you so long?" I said teasingly.

I could see on HER face that I must not have looked very good. Heck, I felt GREAT, compared to a couple hours earlier, but I could tell she was holding back the tears. Later, she admitted that I looked like the **Michelin Man**. I ate the peanuts around 630pm and I was finally released about 2am. She took me home and put me to bed.

* - but didn't realize at the time.

So that's it. The back-story... I had to tell you that so now I can tell you the rest of the story of **living with Peanut Anaphylaxis**.

Chapter 2 - Living with Peanut Anaphylaxis

My safe bubble, my prison

I am a prisoner to this allergy. I live in a bubble where avoidance is possible and safe. I can't leave my bubble without feeling unsafe. I spend too much time and mental energy on avoidance when I'm outside the bubble and it is completely exhausting. If I'm lucky I bring one of my angels with me to keep me safe and sane. Yes, still married to the woman of my dreams, my first angel, 25 years this October.

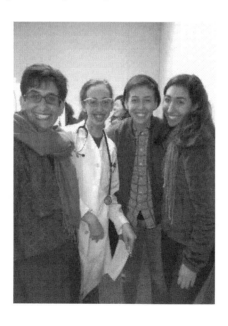

Just last weekend I chose to leave my bubble and tried flying on a new airline because they have some routes that are more convenient for me. It required many hours of preparation and cross checking to make sure that I notified everyone who needed to know about my allergy as well as reconfirming the details. The preparation was time consuming, mentally exhausting and the end result of the travel was less than perfect. But I'm not going back, I'm going forward. I'm going to make this work one way or another.

If you have a kid with LTFA you absolutely need to empower them to advocate for their health and safety so they can avoid, but you should also try to lower their risk. How to do that? I don't know, but for me, I've been waiting 49 long years for something, anything really, just so I don't have to live the rest of my life on 'high-alert' all the time.

Hope is empowering

Immunotherapy (IT) is the process of desensitization by small and progressively increasing exposure to an allergen. The body first develops the ability to tolerate, then long term actually stops reacting to the allergen altogether. This is well established for seasonal and environmental allergies. If you've ever heard of someone being treated with 'allergy shots' this is what they are talking about.

Immunotherapy for food allergies is in its infancy in comparison. It has been proven to be as effective as traditional IT, but it is not without some additional risks due to the anaphylaxis element involved. There are at least four types of immunotherapy. The allergy shots are called subcutaneous or SCIT. SCIT is <u>not</u> being investigated for food allergies.

The IT under investigation for food allergies are:

Oral (OIT) – The allergen is eaten

Sub-Lingual (SLIT) – The allergen is placed under the tongue

Epicutaneous (EPIT®) – The allergen is placed on the skin, a.k.a. 'the patch'

Each of these has shown very promising results but is still considered in the research phase. It will be quite some time before you can get any of these treatments from a major medical health plan. The big healthcare providers won't touch it until it is 'FDA approved'. That could take years.

But there is hope. There are options available today that you can choose to pursue and make your own informed decision on. Understand the risks and benefits, and make the right choice for your circumstances. These are OIT and SLIT. See the Resources section for more information.

Anaphylaxis 101

I grew up before the internet. Publishing back then was expensive. Today, it's practically free and it seems like there are a billion resources on any topic. As a result we are inundated with information. But in addition to the internet, our society has become very litigious, so with every line of advice comes three lines of legal disclaimer. As a result advice from knowledgeable sources gets diluted and suppressed.

Is there a reliable source of information on the free internet? I don't know, but it seems like all the self proclaimed experts tend to parrot each other. Talk about information overload. Should you trust them? No. Should you trust me? Hell NO! The only place to get advice about your medical questions is from your trusted source, usually a doctor, but even they are not infallible or without their own restrictions. **I've nearly died in the 'expert' hands of the medical profession.** *You need to get to the point where you trust YOURSELF.* If you are already there then that is great, now your next step is to transfer that ability to the one with the allergy.

What follows below is what I need to know about Anaphylaxis that enables me to ask more questions if needed.

Signs and Symptoms of Anaphylaxis – www.anaphylaxis101.com

A life-threatening allergic reaction can make someone feel sick in many different ways. While symptoms of an allergic reaction vary from person to person, reactions can quickly progress to become life-threatening – this is called anaphylaxis. It is important to recognize the signs.

The **respiratory** and the **cardiovascular** are the deadly ones. EITHER of those or any TWO of the others is considered anaphylaxis and should be treated as an emergency.

Source: **www.anaphylaxis.ca**

Page 21

SKIN	RESPIRATORY	GASTROINTESTINAL	CARDIOVASCULAR	NEUROLOGICAL
hives, swelling, itching, warmth, redness	coughing, wheezing, shortness of breath, chest pain or tightness, throat tightness, trouble swallowing, hoarse voice, nasal congestion or hay fever-like symptoms, (sneezing or runny or itchy nose; red, itchy or watery eyes)	nausea, stomach pain or cramps, vomiting, diarrhea	dizziness/ lightheadedness, pale/blue colour, weak pulse, fainting, shock, loss of consciousness	anxiety, feeling of "impending doom" (feeling that something really bad is about to happen), headache

OTHER[23]

uterine cramps

When I eat peanuts I experience all five.

> If someone is showing <u>anaphylactic</u> symptoms as described above, from food or otherwise they should be administered using an auto-injector *IntraMuscular* Epinephrine (IM epi) as SOON AS POSSIBLE. If the victim doesn't have the medication on them then ASK EVERYONE. Most likely someone will have one. DON'T WAIT. Administer it in the *outer thigh*, <u>through the clothing</u>, hold in place for 10 seconds, Call 911 and then massage the injection site. With any medication there are risks, but administering <u>one dose</u> and then determining the next course of action is lower risk than not giving the medication. Once the medication is in the system you've bought yourself some time.

Epinephrine doesn't remove the allergen – it merely counteracts the anaphylaxis. You still need to get immediate medical advice and medical attention. Subsequent injections may be needed, or maybe not. If the individual needing the medication is below a certain body weight there is a half- dose auto-injector available.

Disclaimer: In the absence of other medical advice, what's written above is the best I have. Use at your own risk.

Epinephrine Auto-injectors

EpiPen® – The incumbent.
> Largest and was developed for US military.

Adrenaclick® – The alternative.
> About half the size of Epi-Pen.

AuviQ™ – New kid on the block.
> Includes audible instructions.

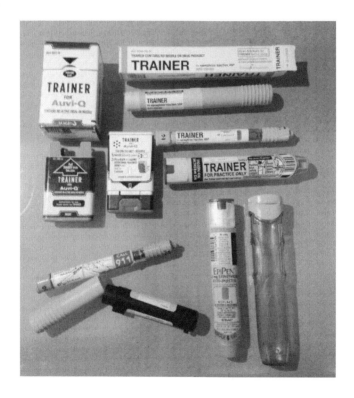

I recently joined the Food Allergy and Anaphylaxis Connection Team (**FAACT**) and in the welcome package they included an AuviQ trainer, so I asked my daughters to use it on me. I gave them no help at all. Let's just say, training on these things is sort of like a fire drill. Everyone knows you should do it, but it never happens. After the AuviQ I pulled out the EpiPen and Adrenaclick trainers and made them do it again. Then I had my wife do it and I tallied up the results. If I was a cat I would have used up more than my nine lives between the all the fake emergencies. Everyone needs to be trained. You can't assume the person that knows what to do will be there when needed.

Everyone needs to be trained.

One last point: It's important to understand the difference between an allergy and anaphylaxis. Please do not use the two terms interchangeably. This is especially important when in discussion with medical professionals during emergency treatment.

IF YOU WANT TO LEARN MORE ABOUT FIRST HAND EXPERIENCES WITH ANAPHYLAXIS AND EPINEPHRINE AUTO-INJECTORS:

- **Eating Peanut: Hesitation:**
http://eatingpeanut.blogspot.com/2014/10/hesitation.html
- **What Anaphylaxis Feels Like**
http://allergistmommy.blogspot.com/2011/11/what-anaphylaxis-feels-like.html
- **Killer Food Allergies:**
https://www.youtube.com/watch?v=XC0nHFblLcE

Allergen Exposure and Allergen Loading

The concept of allergen loading which was explained to me long ago seems to have fallen out of favor. But there have been some **more recent research results** where food allergy sensitivity is increased when the patient also has seasonal (pollen) allergies and those plants are in bloom. For me this is absolutely true.

One of the first lessons learned is that food allergen exposure is not limited to only consumption of the food. Other avenues are:

➢ Contact – on the skin, in the mouth
➢ Inhalation of dust or aerosols – Nasal or lungs
➢ Opthalmic – yes, even on the surface of the eyeball

In most circumstances, the critical element is to remove the allergen exposure if possible. Once eaten or inhaled, there are not a whole lot of options, so the goal is to avoid the allergen in the first place. Use your other sensitivities (sinus or skin) to check first. A contact skin reaction should be cleaned off the skin as soon as possible and once an airborne exposure is determined removal from the environment seems to be the only option.

I've read a **misconception** on the internet on a purported expert site that an airborne reaction is caused by inhalation of allergen which sticks to the esophagus, then is swallowed. This is definitely NOT TRUE and potentially dangerous information. Very little research has been done on this topic, but enough to prove that airborne reactions are real but also proof that there are false positive reactions due to the smell. Just because there are false positives doesn't negate that airborne can also be an exposure path.

When I talk about airborne exposure I am not talking about the SMELL. People can have reactions when they inhale food proteins that they are allergic to. This can occur when food is cooked, when powdered or crushed forms become aerosolized, or in other situations when proteins are released into the air.

The allergic response is to the protein, and pure oil or a pure scent of food alone shouldn't cause a reaction. Regardless, where there is smoke there is fire. I am 'airborne reactive' regardless of the medical explanation. But there is more; when I smell something suspicious it almost always triggers anxiety. Then I have to try to figure out if I'm feeling a legitimate reaction or just the anxiety. Either way, better safe than sorry, so leaving the location where the exposure is occurring is prudent.

True airborne reactions probably depend on the length and concentration of exposure. I am not aware of a death due to airborne, but there are plenty of deaths due to Asthma that uses the same exposure path, so it would seem plausible.

People who are as sensitive as I am instinctively know how to not put themselves at risk. I don't go to bars where the primary snack is peanuts. I don't fly airlines that serve peanuts. I don't go to most Asian restaurants, no professional baseball games; I won't eat in a restaurant where peanuts are in the kitchen. This list goes on and on. If I walk into a room where it doesn't feel right I will leave and here is why:

Even if a reaction doesn't progress to anaphylaxis a minor allergic reaction will cause immediate discomfort and the body will become fatigued as it recovers from the exposure as it eliminates the allergen and replenishes the auto-immune system capabilities. Among true (Food) Allergy sufferers this is referred to the "allergy hangover", and depending on the amount and duration of allergen exposure, it's comparable to a hangover from drinking too much. More on this later.

For skin contact exposure immediate removal with a cleansing (soap) agent is best. Things like hand sanitizer gels don't work. Any cleaning wipe is fine but don't continue to reuse one wipe. The goal is to remove the allergen, not just smear it around.

If it's in the mouth and not swallowed then rinsing out the mouth has always helped me. I have also GENTLY cleaned my mouth with a swab, rag or very soft toothbrush. Be careful not to rub the allergen into the soft tissues of the mouth. At a minimum, rinse and spit, then spit more. I find I get a lot of saliva and mucus at the beginning of a reaction. I've always assumed this is the body's way of ejecting the allergen to minimize ingestion.

The eyes are very sensitive to allergen exposure. In my own experience I've had my eyes swell shut from airborne exposure and I can only imagine that a contact reaction from hand to eye can have the same frightening effect. I've also had my face swell from ingesting the allergen, so it's really difficult to determine the severity or risk of a reaction when it involves their eyes. For this reason my house is absolutely, 100% peanut and tree nut free.

The biggest driver of anxiety in me is simply not knowing how severe a reaction is going to be. All reactions start the same and feel the same. That's why I have a strict avoidance protocol for all food allergens.

More information is in the Resource section at the end. You can also learn more on Facebook: Airborne Anaphylaxis Is Real: A place for sharing stories...

Chapter 3 - Well meant advice

Peanut is not a nut

Although they both have 'nut' in the name, as do other foods that aren't nuts either, peanuts are legumes. Lumping peanuts in with tree nuts leads to confusion that requires further clarification. It's better to just treat them separately: Peanuts (PN) and Tree Nuts (TN). It's possible to be allergic to one without the other. It's also possible to be anaphylactic to one and not the other (like me); hence making this distinction is critical.

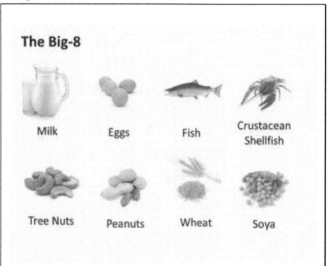

The Big-8

| Milk | Eggs | Fish | Crustacean Shellfish |
| Tree Nuts | Peanuts | Wheat | Soya |

A group of the eight major allergenic foods is often referred to as the Big-8 and comprises **milk, eggs, fish, crustacean shellfish, tree nuts, peanuts, wheat** and **soybean**. These foods account for about 90% of all food allergies in the United States and must be declared on any processed food

> according to the USA food allergen labeling act (FALCPA)[1]. In addition labeling of the Big-8 is mandatory according to EU, Canadian, Japanese and Australian / New Zealand regulations, all of which follow Codex Alimentarius **recommendations**.
>
> **https://farrp.unl.edu/informallbig8**

Explaining your avoidance reasoning: Sometimes it's just the inconvenience

"You can't let your allergy get in the way of your life." I hear that a lot. Sort of like, it would suck if you die, of course, but being overly cautious can 'inhibit' you. Rather than defending my position based on an 'it could kill me', where people look at you funny I started explaining **the major inconvenience that would be caused for myself** and everyone I was with if I took an unnecessary risk. This was actually more effective in diffusing the skepticism over the avoidance protocol. Quite simply:

➢ All allergies start the same with a burning sensation in my mouth. For this reason I also don't eat spicy food. Once the burning starts I have no idea how bad the reaction could be. In general, if you are anaphylactic, the recommendation is 'better safe than sorry'.

➢ This causes me anxiety which coincidentally also has some similar symptoms to anaphylaxis

➢ If I use the IM epinephrine we have to call 911 and that would suck for everyone, and I have to go to the hospital and that's a 2 hour observation once admitted.

➤ If it's a real reaction I will be wiped out for the next several days but I'm supposed to do xx tomorrow and missing that would suck. Then (based on my prior experience) I'd have to be on prednisone for two weeks with all the associated side effects.

➤ Or I could die, now that's unlikely, if the hospital is five minutes away... but what if medical attention is not really that close? Or what if the ER docs don't know what they are doing (based on my prior experience)?

Let me tell you what really inhibits me.

➤ Going out for a social dinner, having a reaction, and spoiling it for EVERYONE. Guess who becomes the social outcast?

➤ You could fly all day anywhere in the world for a series of arranged business meetings that have been scheduled weeks in advance. Try to explain how your carelessness made you miss the meetings. (Never happened to me).

➤ You are on vacation for time with friends and family. Having a reaction will make you miss precious time that can never be recovered.

This is a cute little graphic that really sums it up. On the left is me **if I'm not 100% confident that I will have safe food** between now and when I can get back to my bubble. This could be an afternoon, a weekend or a 2 week business trip in Asia.

32

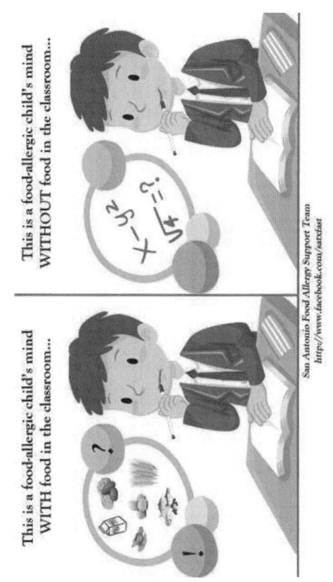

So, in a nutshell here's the most concise reply I give without having to go into detail:

*"I AM HERE TO DO **XXX**. HAVING AN ALLERGIC REACTION RIGHT NOW WOULD PREVENT THAT, SO I'M NOT TAKING ANY CHANCES."*

That's it. No debate, no discussion. Stand strong for your health and safety!

Scorecard (29 year summary)

As best I can remember:

- Two near death experiences (**my back-story**)
- Three major tree nut reactions, not life threatening, but at the time I didn't know for sure. In hindsight I was gambling with my life, but didn't realize it.
- Three 'false alarms', allergen unknown, where I went to the hospital, but by the time I arrived it had passed (did not use epi, that was before the treatment protocol changed)
- One peanut oil --> to hospital, no epi, no anaphylaxis (Boise)
- One peanut oil --> to hospital, used epi (new protocol), no anaphylaxis (Boise (you'd think I had learned??))
- One ER trip for suspected peanut ingestion, turned out to be anxiety and apparently not peanut, since no anaphylaxis. (Ice scream shop)
- Probably several dozen anxiety attacks (roughly three times per year) that were serious enough to interrupt my work or social

plans to the extent it might as well have been a real, non-lethal allergic reaction.

- Hundreds of episodes of anxiety simply for not following my self-imposed avoidance protocols. These were mostly caused by not advocating for myself and eating something that I didn't feel 100% safe about, but in my defense it was different back then. And food labeling wasn't all that wonderful either.

This list does not include any reactions that occurred before my college experience, again, as far as I know those all ended with violent vomiting. Thank God for that.

The inconvenience of a reaction: reality

What follows just showed up recently on Facebook and I've redacted the identities. From the original question to the last comment was about 8 hours. I have never seen a post before where there is not *some* dissention. The response is **UNANIMOUS:**

Original Facebook Post:

I can sleep all day after an [sic] reaction. Is this normal?

Comments:

- It is for me

- I am out of sorts in every way imaginable after a severe reaction.
- I call it the 'allergic reaction hangover'
- Yes! After an allergic reaction, especially if it's severe enough for IV meds, I'm tired for days.
- I do too
- I slept a lot the day after my anaphylactic reaction.
- It is for me.
- Even reactions that aren't ER-worthy wear me out.
- The only time I felt like going to sleep after a reaction was last summer and I had to take a Zyrtec to counteract the reaction I had as a result of something that I ate. After I went to sleep then I felt ok again.
- I pretty much hibernate after a bad reaction. I thinks it's part Benadryl part my body using all it's energy to freak out over whatever I was reacting to
- Yes, the medication only treats the symptoms. your body still needs to get rid of the allergen
- Yeah I'm out of commission for pretty much a week before I start to feel normal again. It's essentially trauma that happens to your body and it needs time to heal
- Yes its not good! Had some wheat earlier that practically knocked me out. It was scary
- My body just feels like it shuts down. I take it to be your immune system in fighting so hard it just knocks you out. I always get fatigued after a reaction.

- I too call it my allergic reaction hangover. It's the worst if I have an anaphylactic reaction, but I still get them from any reaction.
- It would be odd if you didn't.
- I've never had that severe of a reaction food wise but I have however reacted severely to a couple different meds and I ended up feeling that way for days afterwards
- After allergy test my stomach killed me, so took a little children's liq benadryl. Took several days before I felt better and mentally get back to normal.
- could not stop myself from sleeping.

Dining out: Step 1

I was invited to lunch by a fellow who is a vegetarian. It was his turn to choose the restaurant, a place I had never eaten before. It took three email exchanges to get to the answer I was looking for. This information could have easily been on their website along with their menu, they actually have allergy info on their webpage, but nothing specific to peanut.

Imagine having to go through this for every meal that you need to eat and this example was one of the easiest. This is why **I am a prisoner to this allergy.**

Here is the email exchange I had with the restaurant:

From: Me
Subject: Peanut Allergy Info

Do you serve any dishes that contain peanut or peanut oil as an ingredient?

I realize you can't absolutely guarantee me 100% risk free dining, and I accept that risk every moment of every day.

Take a look at this as a reasonable policy as an example: **http://www.united.com/web/en-US/content/travel/specialneeds/needs/peanut-allergies.aspx**

It would save us both time if you could update this document regarding your peanut policy: [redacted]

That way I would not need to email you. And you wouldn't need to respond. <smiley>
Best Regards,

From: Guest Advocate
Subject: RE: Peanut Allergy Info

Hi Michael, We do not have any actual peanuts in the building. The only nuts we have in our restaurants are the ones listed in the doc you have attached. However, some of our boxed items that are delivered to our restaurants contain tree nuts. I hope this helps. Please let me know if you have any other questions. Thanks,

From: Me
Subject: RE: Peanut Allergy Info

Thanks, looking forward to dining with you! Managing this food allergy is a PITA, and I would never consider eating with you had I not been invited by a friend. So, can you address the rest of my email please?

Thanks,

From: Guest Advocate
Subject: RE: Peanut Allergy Info

Michael- To answer your question regarding peanut oil, we use rice bran oil. Thank you!

From: Me
Subject: RE: Peanut Allergy Info

Hi,
Sorry for not being clear. I have a food allergy and it was a lot of work and wasted time for me to determine that your restaurant is OK for me. I would appreciate it if on your website you could provide this information to make my life easier. Do you plan to make any changes to your website based on this suggestion? Thank you!

From: Guest Advocate
Subject: RE: Peanut Allergy Info

Unfortunately, I don't have access to that. However, I can share this information with our team here at the home office. Thanks for your feedback.
Sincerely,

our mission: to provide every guest craveable and convenient veggie-centric food served by a caring, knowledgeable and genuinely engaging Team.

Flying with PA: advice

I have dealt with commercial flights a lot over the years and things have certainly evolved, but even today **no airline will make any guarantee about or controlling the actions of other passengers.** Because I am airborne sensitive I only fly airlines that do not SERVE peanuts themselves.

DISCLAIMER:

> I have actually not flown much since 2010, with **my change in jobs**. I started writing this because I saw a lot of questions on FB, then before I posted I Googled to make sure I wasn't off base. What remains below I believe is still valid and helps you do your own research to support your needs.

Like I said before, I only fly airlines that do not SERVE peanuts themselves. For me that used to be United, Lufthansa, American, and Horizon. You need to check the airline website to get their exact policy. You should also check the published menus if their policy is not explicit. I have had a contact reaction when I was washing out a peanut butter container in college, but no other since so I have flown in an aircraft that has had peanuts served on earlier flights, but maybe I need to rethink that or start taking more precautions (thank you FB). Regardless of the peanut policy on the airlines mentioned or any others I might fly I would never eat anything they serve; only bring your own food which you KNOW is safe. If I had to buy food during travels I would only eat in the airport so if I had a medical emergency I would be on the ground.

Since the mid-'00's I started eating food served by United, however, since revisiting airline policies it seems things have changed quite a bit AGAIN. I could never understand the concept of 'buffer zones' around the allergic individual (but I do now). Airlines that propose buffer zones as a solution don't address airborne exposure. Whenever I'm told *'no one has ever died from airborne exposure on an airplane'* my response is '**and I'm not going to be the first**'.

Once you deal with choosing the right airline how you handle other passengers that bring nuts onboard is your own problem. **Having the allergy announcement is nice, but don't rely on that since the airline cannot legally enforce compliance.** If you fly during peak business travel hours the majority of people **fly all the time and will appear to be annoyed with you, but you can always win them over with either logic or compassion/sympathy**. You know what doesn't work? 1) Being hysterical, 2) calling the flight attendant before you ask them to accommodate you directly.

If you ask them nicely they get to look like a good and helpful person to the people around them, and who doesn't like that? If you call the flight attendant first then you look like a tattletale and they feel like they are getting punished. Furthermore, this persecution complex is compounded if they make the peanut free announcement and you rat them out to the flight attendant because they won't know that it's actually you with the allergy or if you are just being a **buttinsky. Learn to stand strong and advocate for yourself.**

I guess I am only 'moderately' sensitive in comparison and this advice may not work for those who are more sensitive than I. Unfortunately there were **several well documented cases** where communication broke down, assurances were made that could not or would not be kept and someone else came darn close to being the first airborne PN-ANA victim. In summary, in 2013 a woman who knew she was **very** airborne sensitive, flew on United (my preferred airline), they didn't serve any peanuts, but a passenger caused her to go ANA and they made an emergency landing; hospitalization and **lawsuit**.

I would guess this is one reason why policies on this matter have changed in the past year. You can complain all you want about this, but **I would much rather have an airline be perfectly clear about what they will and won't do**, including what they are actually **capable of doing** rather than telling you that it's all in your head and/or 'we will take care of you' when they really won't or can't. I do sympathize that the two families in these two stories flew this airline previously, but apparently United changed their policy and didn't bother to tell anyone.

If you want to rail on the airline industry go to: **http://www.nonuttraveler.com/**

Don't expect an airline to accommodate you **outside of their written policies.** Go to their website and type in the word peanut into the search bar. If what you find doesn't address your concerns, **find another airline**. I use **www.kayak.com** for flight planning but only buy tickets directly from the airline, not through a 3rd party company such as an online travel agent.

Don't expect to wait until the day of the flight at the airport to tell them about your allergies. If you buy the tickets online there may or may not be a way to indicate your allergy so you might have to call to get that noted on your itinerary. Depending on the airline it might be a "fly at your own risk" response. I've experienced the wait time to buy a ticket over the phone might be a few minutes, but the wait time to talk to an agent to add the note to your reservation for free is substantially longer, (like 40 minutes), so buy over the phone and ask all the questions you need to feel comfortable before you commit to buy. If the airline will make any accommodation for you then make sure the allergy needs are noted on the itinerary before the end of the call, which might be in a field that is normally not visible to you. If so, ask them to add a second note that will appear on the printed copy of your itinerary (but not all airlines can do this).

When you are flying you are so far from true medical attention this is one of those situations where strict avoidance is a requirement. As I learned from my earlier reactions epinephrine only lasts so long, and as an adult you have different needs than traveling with your child. Carry 'enough' epi, but how much is really enough??

Becoming your own advocate

I am an **introvert**. If you want to know what that is you can get **this book** or **watch this video**. Dealing with LTFA has been hard medically and emotionally, but the hardest challenge of all was **developing the confidence to be my own advocate.** It would be too complicated or too personal to go through the how I managed to get here, frankly I'm grateful and blessed to be alive. So instead I'm going to tell you the story of someone who truly inspires me. Someone who in 29 months has dealt with more challenges than I dealt with in 29 years. There is one catch however; the story I'm going to tell you is about one of the world biggest **extroverts.** Since this story is a sidebar I will defer back to my blog if you want to read more.

http://peanutoit.com/2015/04/12/becoming-your-own-advocate/

Chapter 4 - Surviving with Peanut Anaphylaxis

Eating out – How to order and eat. When outside your safe bubble (peanut and tree nut example):

What you are about to read may seem excessively cautious to the point of being Obsessive Compulsive Disorder (OCD). I'm sharing it as an example of what I put myself through in order to feel safe when eating out and to feel like I can survive.

1. *Have an angel with you* if at all possible, it makes it so much easier
   a. If you don't have an angel, but have a friend or someone sympathetic to your situation it is 10x more stressful. Even so, if you screw up their meal experience, they aren't going to want to eat with you again. Trust me; it's true, it's happened to me. This is when you learn who your real friends are.
   b. If you are at a business dinner it is 100x more stressful.
   c. If you have a business dinner in a foreign country it is 1000x more stressful.
   d. If you have a business dinner in a foreign country where English is not the primary language it is 10000x more stressful.
2. Pick a restaurant, based on how adventurous you are feeling:
   a. Not very --> go to a safe national chain that you've eaten at before, like fast food, or Pizza

    b. A little --> steakhouse, Italian

    c. Moderate --> Mexican or BBQ

    d. Very --> Something else that I'm not familiar with

    e. Suicidal --> Chinese, Thai. (Just kidding, I never eat here. If invited I decline to go, even to a business dinner.)

3. You are looking to see if there is ANY indication there are peanuts in the kitchen

4. Read the menu outside, if it seems okay then go in

5. Try to get away from the door and near the kitchen if possible

6. Breath! do you smell/sense any sinus reaction?

    a. If not, stay, if so, leave. Unless you can talk directly to either the owner or cook don't bother asking about allergies

7. Get seated, don't touch anything if this is a wipe down establishment, except the menu

8. Read the entire menu in detail, it might not be the same as the one posted outside

9. Look for the 'specials'. (I once went to a safe restaurant that had a special dish with a special ingredient (peanut, of course). Guess what everyone was ordering?)

10. If you see there are any peanuts on the menu or in the kitchen then make sure you order first (most restaurants will customarily want to serve the ladies first) and start with the cross contamination question below.

11. If there is no reason to think there are peanuts in the kitchen then let the waiter do their job as they see fit. No need to go onto extreme alert if there is no risk. You won't enjoy your meal if you can't relax.

Make sure you are dining with people who are not difficult. You should have the most difficult order that they need to take care of and you should be exceptionally nice to the waiter. If they want to take your order across the table I usually ask them to come closer.

12. "I am **deathly** allergic to peanuts and I read your menu and **it looks like you have no peanuts in the kitchen**. Can you confirm that?" If the waiter doesn't have an **immediate** answer and has to check then follow up with the second and third question before they go:

   a. #2 "and please check on peanut oil also"
   b. #3 "and I also allergic to ____, **but it won't kill me**. Please check on those also."
   c. Make sure they write it down before they leave, and then say: "You are going to talk directly to the cook, right?"

13. In my more recent experience the waiter USUALLY has a very clear understanding of these issues and can address the questions on the spot, indicating the restaurant has a clear policy on the matter, in which case if there are no peanuts on the menu there usually aren't any in the kitchen. It's important to feel that the waiter is confident in what they are telling you. Look them straight in the eye and if for a moment you think they don't know either ask them to talk to the cook for you, or ask to speak to the owner, or ask to speak to the cook directly.

14. A good waiter would never want you to circumvent them, so they should be very responsive at this point. The second worst thing that could happen now is for the entire party to

leave, the worst that could happen is that you have an allergic reaction since you were explicitly clear to them and you have a bunch of witnesses. If after all this it looks like from the menu there are no peanuts, but it turns out that there actually are then you should ask to talk to the manager on duty or the owner regarding this hazard and the implications on whether or not you stay. Explain the situation and that it would be helpful to you and people like you if the menu could be more explicit. [This has not happened to me recently, but it used to a lot.] At this point if your anxiety will prevent you from enjoying the meal thank the waiter and leave.

15. If you think you might want to stay then go to the cross contamination questions below.

16. Cross Contamination:
    a. "I see you have dish(es) with peanuts. I am deathly allergic to peanuts. How well does your kitchen manage cross contamination?"
    b. If in a Mexican or BBQ restaurant:
    c. "I am deathly allergic to peanuts. Does your mole, enchilada or BBQ sauce have peanuts in it?"
    d. Northern Mexican style - probably Yes
    e. Southern Mexican style - Probably No -- >> If yes, follow up with the cross contamination question.

17. If you are satisfied with the response then ask about peanut oil and inform the waiter about all other non-ANA food allergies and ask if those will be a problem. If you are satisfied with all the answers and even if you completely trust what they are telling you **it is still OK to leave if you aren't going to enjoy the meal.** If you decide you

are still ok with eating in a restaurant with peanuts then indicate the others at the table can order. This will give you time to de-stress and decide what you want. Take a deep breath and try to relax; you've passed the first gauntlet.

> The last time I chose to stay in a restaurant with peanuts in it we almost had a fantastic meal and no one at our table ordered food with peanuts, but unfortunately the adjacent table did. I had a few bites before they were served, but I am not able to bring myself to eat anything if I can smell peanuts. Because I had grilled the waiter and they had passed my test I thought it would be unreasonable for me to make a stink about it. I was there, it was my choice, and I knew the risk. I didn't finish my meal and went outside to get some fresh air. Lesson learned. Had this been a business dinner I probably would have stayed and had the waiter clear my plate. Sitting there and not eating the food in front of you makes your fellow diners uneasy.

18. Now, time to order. You cannot order ANYTHING that is deep fried, you have no idea what else went in that fryer. Choose a meal that is the most bland and safest option on the menu. Ask for all sauces and dressings on the side. The waiter will look at you like you are nuts, like "you just gave me the 3rd degree over the menu and kitchen and you're ordering that??" And when you are done ordering, remind them that it is a very serious allergy. When they bring you your food the server should repeat back

everything special about the order, or give some sort of blanket guarantee that they double checked with the cook and there are no allergens in your meal.

19. Now, to eat. If by chance anyone else has ordered what you ordered wait for them to eat first and assess whether or not the food is safe. If you have any concerns about your own food ask the angel to taste test for you. Try to 'smell' the food, but when I take anti-histamines for seasonal allergies this doesn't always work.

20. Start with the sauces and dressings, dip one tine of your fork in the sauce and dab it on your lip. Depending on your sensitivity to the allergen wait long enough before doing the next. Decide which item you want to eat first and break off a tiny piece, chew, but don't swallow (I usually start with the steamed vegetables.) Hold it in your mouth long enough to determine if it is safe, if not, or if there is any question, cough or sneeze into your napkin and SPIT IT OUT. If you have any concern ask your angel to taste test for you Because of my prior experience and belief that a full stomach will delay onset of a reaction I'm in the habit of eating all of one item at a time, starting with the safest.

21. Never mix, and pause between items long enough to ensure there is no reaction. I do all this very discretely and no one can tell, except my angels, if someone asks me if I don't like the food they also run interference for me.

22. After completing the main courses successfully and feeling at ease you may be tempted to eat dessert.

23. WHAT ARE YOU NUTS?? **Dessert is the most dangerous item on the menu!** Usually from an outside bakery. Don't tempt fate. You had a good outcome, don't screw up now. If your waiter took good care of you tip them AT LEAST 20%. If you aren't paying the bill then slip them some cash for taking care of you. **This whole experience is merely a trial run for the next time you come back here to order what you really want.** Exhausted yet? I am, just thinking about it, but you still have the burden of deciding if this restaurant is any closer to moving into your safe bubble.

Call me crazy if you want, but my last anaphylactic reaction was in 1987.

Airborne Allergy Discovery at 36,000 feet

My father owned his own contracting business in Detroit and insisted all his kids go to college and get a 'white-collar' job. I ended up with an engineering degree and went to Silicon Valley in the high tech field. I worked for a large multi-national company, but didn't realize that in order for my career to progress would require business travel. Some times more than others, both domestic and international, but YIKES!! What did I get myself into?

When I started flying the attendants pushed peanuts out with every drink. Slowly there was conversion to non-peanut snacks. It was a nuisance, but not horrible, and my initial travels were domestic flights. Back then the climate control systems brought in more fresh air from the outside so I would blow the air vent on my face wide open to avoid 'smelling' the peanuts. On today's more modern aircraft the ventilation systems are more energy efficient, bring in less outside air and recirculate it more. The modern aircraft have HEPA filters, and **if they are working properly** should remove the airborne allergens, but the catch is that not 100% of the air is filtered every time it passes through.

In the early '90's I was flying to Dallas on **American Airlines** and one of the two menu choices was a dish swimming in peanut sauce. Everyone was served and uncovered their food and I went into what I would describe as a very serious hay fever type reaction, sneezing, watery & swollen eyes but <u>much</u> worse than my typical seasonal allergies. I had never been through this before. I had the Ana-kit out and I hit the call button for the flight attendant. I told her what was going on and she immediately cleared the used plates away around me as quickly as possible. I could feel my face swelling and my eyelids getting pushed closed. I didn't use the epi. Fortunately the portions were small and eaten quickly and the fresh air was blowing on my face. The reaction went away almost as quickly as it came on, but from that time on I always called the airline in advance to confirm the menu to make sure there would be no peanuts in the meal. Apparently that dish was not very popular and so I never encountered it again. At some point **United Airlines declared themselves peanut free** and American came close to making the same policy, so these have been my 2 preferred airlines ever since, and both have hubs at the major airport nearest me. I've flown others, provided they were safe by the criteria posted previously.

Flying with PA: Customer service hell

False sense of security

I had become complacent since I only flew 'safe' airlines. In 2008 I booked a vacation to Israel with a tour group and the airline ticket was included. I failed to check at the time which airline it was. After the ticket was booked I read their peanut policy and immediately tried to get out of flying with them. I called and explained my situation and asked for a refund so I could fly a different airline. **They refused, and told me I would be fine.** I was foolish and meek. I hadn't had a reaction in years and my flying had been completely uneventful, so I let myself be talked into it. I thought they would be handing out those little bags of peanuts, and I was able to deal with those years before, and they 'generously' were providing a buffer zone around me. But that's it, and no announcement either, but I thought nothing of it. We were flying about five hours cross country then going trans-Atlantic. It was a very large, wide body aircraft and I was about 8 or 10 rows behind the end of the first class cabin. The main cabin was divided in half front to back with over wing exits and a curtain between. We were in the air and I was expecting them to offer 'pretzels or peanuts' in little packages. But oh no, the cart coming down the aisle was loaded to the gills with every imaginable peanut based snack for sale. Cookies, candy bars, big bags of peanuts and my anxiety went through the roof.

I just kept telling myself no one ever died from airborne in an airplane. But the little voice inside my head kept telling me 'and I don't want to be the first.' Then it occurred to me... it's not just about me, I'm not the only one affected by this. I thought of my wife, my kids, my family and friends. Did I want to prove myself a going down in the history books as the first person to die on an airplane from airborne exposure, **or did I want to LIVE?**

The cart was coming closer and closer. People were tearing open their snacks, I could start to sense the airborne peanut dust and we were thirty minutes into a five hour flight. Finally, the cart was at the buffer zone, it was in **my 'safety zone'**. At least they would stop serving the peanuts, then the cart would go by and I could go talk to the head flight attendant, or so I thought.... BUT... they kept serving the peanut snacks. **They weren't honoring the buffer zone that they promised me.** I waited until the nice lady came by and when I declined to purchase a peanut snack she smiled and slipped little free bag of peanuts into my hand. That was all I needed. I stood up and said

"Excuse ME" ...

How I got to the front of the aircraft is not clear. But I knew I could not appear to be hysterical, they would dismiss me as having anxiety, and I would go down in history, but not in the way I wanted. I was up front talking to the head attendant, I was calm on the outside but I could feel my heart pounding, as I outlined my grievance and the dire situation:

1. I had spoke to customer service several times weeks and months prior to the flight trying to get out of it, but they assured me I would have no

problem on the flight and would not refund my ticket as requested. They were wrong and **now I was having an airborne reaction.**

2. I was promised me a buffer zone, but that did not happen, as evident by the bag of peanuts in my hand, and it was not clear if anyone onboard knew about my allergy or the buffer zone since it was violated. I spoke to the gate agent prior to the flight and was assured the flight crew would be informed of the allergy and buffer zone. I made this point very clear to the head attendant.

3. I brought my epi-pens, but if I needed to use them they would be required to make an emergency landing at the first possible opportunity. I was insistent on this point. *I doubt they would accommodate this request today. This is one thing that seems has changed with the increased awareness of the PA ANA and airlines are putting the burden of responsibility back on the passenger.*

4. I also asked them to increase the amount of external air in brought into the cabin to clear out the allergens but I was told on modern aircraft like this that is no longer a capability they can control.

I was standing in the first class galley and I had the potential for a great audience (witnesses, should my family need to sue for a wrongful death). My next step at this point would be to back into the first class cabin and repeat it all so that everyone within earshot heard every word. I thought that none of the business travelers would want the plane to have to land because of me. I didn't have to actually do that, but I was getting ready to. I was a little surprised how long it took to finally agreed to stop serving peanuts ... **but only in my section.** I told them no, **it had to be in the whole airplane,** since they had just told me about the air circulation and lack of fresh air. They could not serve any peanuts in the whole airplane. To which they finally agreed. I was relieved that they stopped the peanut service before completing it, and then **announced AN APOLOGY to everyone who didn't get their goodies**. I was at the time surprised they didn't also call me out by name or seat number as the villain of this travesty.

I hung out in the galley for a while because I thought the air was fresher. Eventually they asked me to return to my seat. I had managed to keep my anxiety in check until I sat down. If they THOUGHT this was anxiety driven they would discredit my concerns. I went back to my seat and tried to calm down, but I couldn't. I took Benadryl at some point, might have been before talking to the flight attendant, but I was panicking about a reaction that could come on as quickly as **my previous experience** from the allergens that I had already been exposed to. About 30 minutes later I can't take the anxiety any more so I found someone in our travel group who I thought was a doctor and he talked me down. I returned back to my seat again and tried to rest and figure out what I needed to do for the next leg of this journey. A few hours later I had to go forward and talk to the head attendant again.

"I'm having a reaction to peanuts" I tell her. "I thought you said they would not serve any in the whole aircraft?"

She had a puzzled look and picked up the phone to the aft cabin and after confirming my suspicion she told them to stop immediately. Yes, in fact they had started serving the peanut snacks in the back of the aircraft, behind the curtain where I couldn't see it but the ventilation system had brought it forward to my location. **I was furious.**

The next leg of the journey

We landed and I went to customer service, restated the original complaints and described the omissions on the flight I had just finished. I insisted that they put me on a different airline. They stonewalled me. They kept re-reading their peanut policy to me over and over again.

"They could not guarantee that passengers wouldn't have peanuts on the flight, they couldn't guarantee that the cabin was free from trace residue of peanuts, SO, **because of that** *why couldn't they also serve peanuts during the flight?*"

My favorite, and I even included it in my letter to the president of the airline, was from the gate chief:

"Every airline that flies to Tel Aviv serves peanuts"

They just didn't get it. I just fell back on the "I asked you to refund my ticket and you refused, and you assured me I would be safe, but that didn't happen" so I was not going to back down. I was not going to risk 10 hours exposure in an aircraft, over the middle of the ocean. I wouldn't board the aircraft until I got the assurances I wanted. No peanuts served at all during the whole flight. I was the last passenger left to board. If I didn't board the plane they would be required to find my luggage and remove it (post 9-11 requirement). This could delay the flight considerably. It was a standoff. Finally they agreed. The gate crew told me there would be no peanut service, and that would be OK **"because it was a red-eye flight and the other passengers wouldn't miss it too much."** **OMFG**! I walked down the jet way and stood at the door of the airplane.

"I need to speak to the person in charge of the cabin."

Nothing...

"I'm not boarding until I speak to the person in charge of the cabin."

The purser finally shows up and introduces himself.

I said, "when I boarded the plane in San Francisco the gate crew assured me that they had informed the flight crew about my situation, but apparently that didn't actually happen. So before I step on the plane you need to tell me exactly why I'm standing here and what you will be doing for me on this flight."

The answer that I got was satisfactory.

The flight was uneventful. I arrived and felt sick. There was one photo that I have of me in the Tel Aviv airport, my face was bright red and my eyes were bloodshot. Not sure if it was the stress, lack of sleep, residual allergen exposure or all of the above. I slept the next day through and the day after I saw a doctor who prescribed me some antihistamines and Valium. So before even starting the vacation I had already lost 2 days out of 14. On the 3rd day I called the travel insurance people telling them that they needed to put me on a different flight, but that wasn't covered under their policy. I had never bought travel insurance before and have not since, what a waste. I bought a one way ticket home on Lufthansa/United.

The vacation included a gourmet dining plan, but I was so traumatized based on what had happened on the flight that I limited my food to white bread, goat cheese, fresh fruit and hard-boiled eggs. These were the only foods I could feel were absolutely safe and free from any possible cross-contamination.

THE SEA OF GALILEE:

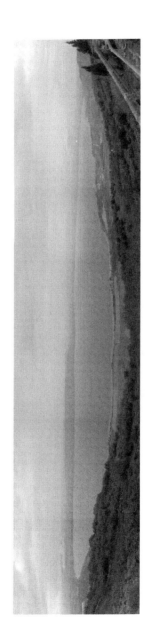

Whenever any of my fellow travelers encouraged me to try some other food I fell back on:

"I'm here to experience being in the Holy Land. If I have an allergic reaction I'll miss out on that, so I'm not taking any chances."

Getting home

I went to the airport for my new flight which departed about 8 hours after the rest of the tour. I said goodbye about 8pm and their flight took off about 10pm. I could not go through security until the following workday. There were no seats or benches outside. All the shops were closed. I circled the Tel Aviv airport pushing my luggage cart until 4am. Finally, I got to go up to security hoping to get through and rest before boarding the aircraft. I had been awake for about 20 hours and I'm sure I did not look all that wonderful. They asked me to step into an office off to the side with my luggage. They asked me:

"Why are you not flying with the rest of your tour group?"
"Why do you have two plane tickets back to the US?"

When I saw the doctor in Jerusalem I had him write me a note on his letterhead stating that I was not to return home on the same airline that brought me due to the risk of peanut exposure. I also showed them my EpiPen and Israeli prescriptions that corroborated my story. They searched my luggage anyway because they probably thought I was a suicide bomber. In hindsight I'm surprised it wasn't a strip search.

After spending a wonderful time with friends in an amazing place I was quite lonely flying home alone, but when I boarded the aircraft I took a deep breath and the air felt safe, like stale cigarette smoke, but peanut free. At least I rested on those flights.

So I guess the gate chief was wrong, there are flights to Tel Aviv that don't serve peanuts.

Epilogue: Customer Service Hell

After I got home I gathered all the documentation, including call records the phone company and was planning to sue the airline in small claims court. I spoke to an attorney friend who agreed to help. First, he had me write a letter to the airline and outline my grievances and claim. When I got no response he wrote a letter on his letterhead informing them he was representing me and I would be suing. That finally got a response. My claim was turned over **to some secret department that no one knows about**. It's their job to make problems go away as cheaply as possible. They didn't want a lawsuit. My friend advised me that they were NOT going to settle because of the allergy, or the anxiety, or the inconvenience caused. Rather **they were going to settle for three reasons and only three reasons:**

1. they made certain promises to me, then failed to keep those promises

2. I had a legitimate LTFA and medical problem (not the anxiety) because of #1 and saw a doctor at my own expense because of it, had his note and had receipts for the cost of the change in travel plans.

3. I had documented proof for both #1 and #2.

Without all three I wouldn't stand a chance, and regardless the settlement would not include pain/suffering/inconvenience.

I was excited when they made me the settlement offer, since I thought this was the beginning of a negotiation, and I wanted to fight for more, but I was advised by the attorney to take the offer and put it behind me. He said they wouldn't negotiate with me directly, only through him, and I took it to mean that his pro bono services were no longer available. So I took the offer. It covered about 50% of the cost of the 2nd flight home. I submitted the medical expense to my health insurance and got a partial reimbursement per my policy,

I vowed to never fly them again...

Bad Doggy Kisses

Facebook is like a cocktail party, lots of conversation, but it disappears in a blur. I love it and I hate for almost the same reason. I have been following lately, trying to learn, trying to educate. Turns out you are never too old to learn something new, like:

- some dogs eat treats with peanuts or peanut butter
- dogs groom themselves, may have peanut on their fur

I learned this reading Facebook. Imagine that, something truly useful!

Peanut was never an issue with our previous dog who lived to be 17, he was a 20 pound terrier and a homebody, spoiled rotten by the kids and I'm sure he thought he was one of them. He was a mutt but best of all however, he was **the only other boy in the house**, and I needed a wingman sometimes. We'd walk him on a leash, but never socialized with other dogs and never traveled with us. So no peanuts for him and no other dogs in our life.

When we finally decided it was time to get another we agreed we wanted a dog that could go to the park and fetch, should be short hair and thin coat so not shed so much. We also thought with the kids growing up that we should get 2 dogs to keep each other company, and these two dogs should be not more than 70 pounds combined weight.

150 pounds of doggy love

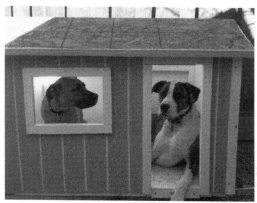

Well, we met two of the three criteria. Of course our dogs are peanut free, but we take them shopping to the pet store, they sometimes need to go to the dog wash and many mornings I run them to a park where they can go off leash and frolic with other dogs. I always have my epi auto-injector with me if I plan on eating anything, but for some reason jogging was a time when I felt OK without it.

The other dogs at the park are friendly and I often pet them, but what really hit home happened just recently. I was giving a scratch to an older Scottie who likes the attention, and a new puppy decided she wanted in on the act, so I'm squatting down and she runs up to me, puts her paws on my shoulders and give me a big, wet, French kiss. At the time I thought nothing of it, but by the time I got home I had put two and two together. ... That could have been a bad situation.

So from now on, I'm going to start bringing my EpiPen and my phone where ever I go.

Chapter 5 - There is one question that you should NEVER ask

People are well intentioned and they want to help keep you safe. You need to **help them help you**. You don't need to ask them lots of questions, but rather ask them the right questions. There is however one question you should never ask. That question is "**Is this safe?**" Let me tell you why.

You are looking for the answer to the question "Is it safe?", but ultimately **only you can answer that for yourself**. When you ask that question to someone else you are effectively **putting the burden of your safety on them**.

If you are talking to a person what they hear is "**If I die, it will be your fault.**" If you are talking to a mom and pop restaurant owner you are saying "**I might give you a bad yelp review**" and if you are talking to an airline you are saying "**I'm going to sue for as much as possible.**"

That individual that you might be unintentionally burdening probably has enough problems of their own without you adding to it, **so don't do it.** They are either doing their job or running their business and just trying to get by like the rest of us. You need to help them help you. You also need to decide what is more important, **your satisfaction or your safety?**

Corporations are not people

Did you read their corporate policy? **No employee has the authority to change that**, so don't ask them to. If you really complain enough they will tell you buy from another company. Are they discriminating against you because of the allergy? No, they are not. They don't want to serve you **because you are asking them to make an exception to the written policy.** Is this legal? YES, IT IS.

The Food Industry

Food cross-contamination is based on the facility where it is produced and NOT the brand. The labeling on the package is specific to the factory. The same item from two different factory locations could have different allergen risks. You could reside in an area where your local store carries the same item from different factories, maybe not at the same time, but might switch unexpectedly from safe to unsafe temporarily or permanently.

This is why YOU HAVE TO READ THE LABELS ON EVERY PACKAGE EVERY TIME. No exceptions.

Airlines

Airlines? Why write about airlines? Why are airlines so important? One simple word, "Airborne". I'm not just referring to being locked in a sealed container with potential allergen exposure from which you can't escape. I'm also referring to the fact that you are FAR from true medical attention.

Based on what I read on Facebook, seem to be that certain airlines seem to be deliberately putting rude/insensitive people in customer facing positions in order to discourage us from flying with them. This to me is sad, because United was the first airline to go 100% peanut free and to this day probably provides the safest environment for Peanut Anaphylaxis. Everyone loves Delta and Southwest lately because they have great customer service, but, you realize you are entering an enclosed environment where peanuts have been recently. **Is that really safe? ... Only you can answer that question.**

You want the airline to make an emergency landing? **It's NOT going to happen anymore.** That's why the policies have changed recently, and you can't afford to sue them.

Unless you have the basis of material financial damage (i.e. loss of breadwinner or extra travel expenses) you don't have a case, and if you are out a few thousand $ for changes in travel plans it will cost you more in legal fees to sue them than you will get.

The employees are under pressure to get the plane back in the air quickly. If the airplane is not flying then it's not making money. I'd also guess the airlines have had plenty of complaints from non-allergic passengers that WE somehow inconvenience them. I'd sure like to know what happens when there is an unplanned emergency landing. How many complaints do they get when that happens? What is the true financial cost to the airline?

All the profit from a flight comes from premium seats. They fill the economy seats just to cover their operating costs. So when you have dozen or more highly paid business execs, the airlines most profitable customers, diverted due to an emergency landing, making them miss their 'important' meetings who do you think they listen to? Us, the 1-2% needy allergic people, or the people **that pay** 2x to 10x what we pay in order to not mingle with the 'riff-raff'? And if you are sitting in first class because you got an upgrade using frequent flyer miles you don't count. There is a little code on your ticket that says so. This is one situation where money talks the loudest.

Take the Erin Brockovich story. All about the collective damage, nothing about the one individual that has an unfortunate accident. **Don't set yourself up to be that accident,** you will be better off by not having the accident in the first place. When dealing with corporations I put my safety above their customer service.

People are People

Now that we've got the corporations behind us let's talk about the people. Years ago I was helping someone refinance their mortgage. I appealed to the broker by telling him the person I was helping was a widowed, retired school teacher. The broker cut me short and told me **"everyone has a sob story; this is what I can do for you today."** He basically told me to stop wasting his time. If you want people to help you:

- get their attention
- tell them exactly what you need
- let them do their job
- don't waste their time

Start with the high level questions and only if necessary get into the details. Despite the severity of my allergy it is actually easy to manage because my requirements are so specific and I'm perfectly clear on what I need. I sympathize with those that have more complex issues to manage. But you can get people to do their best if you help them help you.

- Visit the company website to see if they have a policy on the issue you need addressed. Employees will not be able to override corporate policy, so don't show up and expect them to. **It's all about liability and if they break the rules they can be fired.**
- Contact the company before you arrive to determine what they can answer in advance versus when you arrive. If they tell you they can't accommodate then look for another solution.
- When you arrive make sure you are talking to the person responsible for answering your questions. For example, at a restaurant that would be the waiter, the cook and the manager/owner. Don't bother the host/hostess or the busboy. They aren't allowed to answer these questions even if they want to because they don't handle your food, it's a liability issue.

ADVOCATE

Sometimes you need to lead off with a really clear statement:

- I realize you can't absolutely guarantee me a 100% risk free environment, and I accept that risk every moment of every day, but I need to know ...
- I only fly airlines that do not SERVE peanuts themselves.
- I am here to do XXX. Having an allergic reaction right now would prevent that, so I'm not taking any chances.
- I am deathly allergic to peanuts and I read your menu and it looks like you have no peanuts in the kitchen ...

Side Effects ... and a whole lot more

If it is not already apparent I am being treated for clinical anxiety over the LTFA. My goal is to go through IT in order to eliminate the anxiety and ultimately get off the medication. In the meantime I been getting caught up on **the TV show** "*Once ... upon a time*. It's a great show and family friendly, and it's on ABC, so no premium channel required. I'm watching it with my teenage daughter; what a great bonding experience. We get to talk about good vs. evil, bullying, respect, truthfulness, prince charming and how to find true love. **I've never had a more engaged discussion with her about things that really matter in life**, like whether Regina is evil or good and why? How did she get this way? It's a great story with deep character development. Think of it as a mash-up of **Grimm's Household Tales**, the play '**Into the Woods**' and **Disney's fairy tales** plus **a** whole lot more! What I mean regarding this TV show is that there are a whole bunch more stories woven in that don't originate from the three bases listed above. Pretty awesome!

The consistent two messages of the show is

ALL MAGIC, EVEN GOOD MAGIC, COMES WITH A PRICE

Whoa!! ... These hits a little too close to home. Sort of like these meds I'm taking. The price you pay is the side effect.

And

TRUE LOVE IS MORE POWERFUL THAN MAGIC

My goal is to get off the meds someday, but I can't do it alone. Fortunately I have my family to watch over me. With them I can learn to address the LTFA. **Immunotherapy has given me hope that it can be done.** Just two years ago I was resigned that it was hopeless. Two months ago things had turned around completely and were looking great, then...

TWO WEEKS AGO I DISLOCATED MY JAW.

Oh, the irony. I'm moving down this path so I can eat and live without anxiety but the med I am using to help me along has now prevented me from chewing. **The meds come with a price, just like magic.**

Teeth clenching is a side effect and is the reason why I dislocated my jaw. It's probably been going on since January, but I assume that one night I slept funny with my jaw pushed to the side and when I woke up I couldn't close my mouth, couldn't chew and it was pretty painful. I tried to get it to heal without changing meds, but that wasn't going to work so onto a new one. This is just a minor setback. I am still full of hope.

This is the 4th different med I've tried; I was on the 3rd the longest. Soon moving to #5. Can't wait to see how this new one is going to affect me. Just like allergies everyone is different and has different needs. Some medications are great for some, but for others, not so much.

So, what's the big deal about medication? Nothing I suppose, if it would do what it says it will, but in my experience that has never been the case. There has always been some unintended consequence, a side effect or an artifact. Whether it's aspirin, ibuprophen, anti-histamines, you name it, there is always some short or long term side effect. Even epinephrine has some risks that begin when you get older.

My goal is to address the cause, not just treat the symptoms.

Chapter 6 - Protecting the ones we love

Last week I received in the mail a medical alert bracelet that I bought from Handmade by Heroes. It's not the most high tech option out there, and it's not the cheapest, but it gets the job done. Isn't that all that really matters?

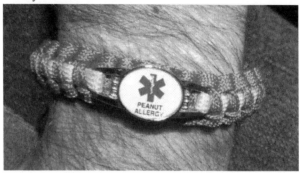

I don't wear jewelry because my skin reacts to metals. This cord is pliable nylon and has an optional plastic clasp. Protect the ones you love and at the same time help out the vets that have risen to the call in defense of our nation. Safe guarding our rights comes at a cost and ultimately the biggest price is paid by men and women serving in our armed forces.

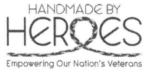

HANDMADE BY
HEROES
Empowering Our Nation's Veterans

No remuneration was received for this endorsement. It's my honor to wear this.

Insulin Angel Medication Tracker

I think the **Insulin Angel medication tracker** is a great idea and there is no reason why it cannot be used for Epinephrine auto-injectors. **It warns you if your cell phone and your meds become separated and continuously tracks the temperature.** The expiration of a medication **depends significantly on the temperature**, in addition to time elapsed. This will help identify if it's potentially gone bad* before expiration and if used properly will extend the life expectancy of meds stored at a more benign temperature. The cost of this device is paid for if the 'expiration' of the epi is extended by just a few months. I started carrying epi in 1986, and the expiration time back then was definitely longer than 1 year. I'm sure they brought it down to reduce their liability in a lawsuit, but also ... **to get everyone to throw away perfectly good meds and buy new.**

Here's the **journal article**:
http://www.annallergy.org/article/S1081-1206(15)00046-0/abstract

FOOTNOTE:

*- Gone bad caused by leaving new epi in a hot car. At the time the liquid was clear, but turned brown months well within the expiration date.

The Indigogo fundraiser is now closed. You can find out more at: **http://www.insulinangel.com/**

Veta Smart Case for Epi-pen

The Veta™ is a Smart case for remote monitoring of your child's Epi-pen.

https://www.youtube.com/watch?v=4-eIQIayeUw

➤ **Veta™** connects loved ones and caregivers to people living with life-threatening allergies, resulting in increased freedom, security and confidence for everyone involved. The Veta system includes:

➤ Veta smart case, which holds your EpiPen®

➤ Veta app, running on iPhone®, iPad®, iPod touch® and Android™ mobile devices, connecting to your support networks through a cloud-based infrastructure.

https://www.aterica.com/product/veta-2/

Recommendations are merely recent observations of innovative products intended to keep us safer. No compensation was received; this is just what I stumbled upon recently.

Chapter 7 - My OIT Story, the beginning

I am not a liar, but ... "Fluid replenishment or Hypotension?"

This was one criteria for exclusion from the clinical study. Jeez, that was almost 30 years ago, and at the time, I didn't remember it in completely vivid detail. OK, yes, they gave me an IV, sure, but do I remember why? The memory can do funny things, especially when there is emotional trauma involved. "Fluid replenishment or Hypotension?" If I check the "yes" box will they eliminate me? ... Wait a minute; I went to the informational meeting. I met the guy that was the success story. He was going to the hospital all the time, now he's eating 17 peanuts a day. They took him in the study. Surely he was hypotensive, right? I mean, you can't be anaphylactic and not be hypotensive, right? I could have been him. I could be eating 17 peanuts a day. But I'm not. I shouldn't have hung up the phone.

I read about Phase 1 of the study a few years earlier and thought my dreams had been answered. I called the number, hoping for a wonder drug treatment. I was ecstatic when they called me back, and I fit the profile, but then they said, "It's quite simple really, we are going to **feed you minute amounts of peanuts**" and I hung up the phone. I didn't even say goodbye, I just hung up the phone. The feeling of hope quickly washed away as my heart raced and anxiety chilled me. Now years later Phase 2 recruiting started. I had plenty of time to think about it. Did I make a mistake? No, I didn't. Sure I'd like to think I could be that guy eating 17 peanuts a day, but fact of the matter is there is no way I could have made it through the peanut exposure; I had spent 25 years reprogramming my anxiety response into a warning system. I had training myself that if I'm anxious I don't eat. I wasn't going to be able to reverse that overnight.

I didn't see the silver lining at the time, but shortly thereafter there was a major restructuring at work and I was on the wrong side of a political power struggle. I was put in a very stressful work environment that turned into a vicious cycle of anxiety and depression that fed on itself relentlessly. I was asked to leave. I was not ready to leave, but I had to. When I sought treatment for this temporary situation the doctor unwound what I had been doing, using anxiety as my warning system. "Anxiety will kill you, **just as dead as eating a peanut,** but it will take a lot longer" And so began my treatment for LTFA induced anxiety.

By the time Phase 2 came around I was ready. I could manage my anxiety. I needed this treatment. I needed to be part of the clinical trial. I was ready to be part of the clinical trial, and frankly, I was desperate. At least if I died during the trial I would know that I had tried my best. I was willing to accept that consequence. And so for the box marked "Fluid replenishment or Hypotension?"

I checked the box next to the *NO*.

Work Life Balance

I was working hard and doing well the first five years at my last job. I had three beautiful daughters, and in my free time enjoyed working with my hands. I enjoyed building things. I enjoyed creating. I fixed things around the house and when I went to cocktail parties all the other men there would pull me aside and tell me that I'm making them look bad. But something was missing. I needed something for me. Something more social. My friend and former work associate invited me to his Tuesday night poker game. It was Texas Holdum and I had never played before, so something new to learn. I was never that good at the game, but it was relaxing to be around others. I learned the rules of poker, how to deal, how to bet and betting strategies, One of the rules was that when you made a bet **it was mandatory that you verbally stated what you were doing** in case you accidentally threw in too many or too few chips. I learned why in professional tournaments some players wear hats with large bills and some wear mirrored glasses, and why you should never ever touch your chips unless you are betting, and some keep their hands below the edge of the table.

You don't want to tip off the other players when you are bluffing. If you do it unconsciously it's called a 'tell'. And I thought I learned all about bluffing, all about **how not to have a 'tell'**. This was useful stuff; I was an engineer by education, but working in sales. Poker was a great experience for me. I went for about a year but then something came up at home, an opportunity to create something out of nothing, I built a loft in my attic since three girls in one bedroom was getting kind of cramped. It took all my spare time for an entire summer. So I put poker night on hiatus, and ultimately never went back because although it was social it wasn't giving me everything that I needed at that point in my life.

A few years later

I was working with a new person in the sales department and it was absolutely wonderful. It was like she could read my mind and yet we worked together only over the phone or by email. I tried to figure out how she was doing that but she never told me. Finally we were at the annual sales conference and after dinner and some wine I confronted her again about her super-power.

"It's easy", she said, "Whenever it's important I can hear it in your voice."

I was dumbstruck. All that time playing poker and **I had a TELL in my voice**!

Job Change

On an unrelated matter there was a restructuring at work a few years later and they wanted me to stay. I tried to stay, to prove myself, but in the back of my mind I thought I wasn't doing too well and I became anxious. In hindsight I wasn't anxious about losing my job, I was anxious about the thought of being forced out of the safe bubble that I had taken 11 years to build. Ironically, it became a self fulfilling prophecy. The anxiety consumed me, I couldn't do my job, and they fired me because I wasn't doing my job. I would have fired me too. **I don't blame them** (anymore), and I've given up the thought of going back, because **I no longer need to.**

Clinical Trial Acceptance Testing

Interview

The interview was pretty much a recap of the written application and establishing rapport with the clinic. I only lied on one question, otherwise, completely honest. After the interview and signing the release forms for admittance testing the first step is confirmation the allergy is real. This is done with a skin test. They applied six allergens to my skin and waited.

I'm cured

Yep, my happy ending. I didn't react to peanuts. I must have grown out of it. I had mixed feelings about this. Wouldn't it be great to not worry anymore? But if so, then how long have I been **torturing** myself unnecessarily?? But wait, not only did I not react to peanuts, but not to pollen or dust mites or mold. **I am superhuman!** The doc looked at my arm and asked if I had been taking any antihistamines in the last 7 days. Of course not, they told me not to and I didn't. He said "you didn't react to **that one**, that's pure histamine, **everyone reacts to that one.**" Then he looked something up on the computer. "It seems the medication you are taking has an anti-histamine side effect." **Oh, the irony!** The anxiety medication I'm taking **because of the PN ANA** is going to eliminate me from the potential **cure for PN ANA!** Then he went off to consult with others.

> Histamine is the control; it's there to prove the test is valid. Just like this skin test a clinical trial needs a control group too, to prove the trial is valid. In this trial 20% of the participants would be in the control group that means 20% are given pure placebo and are not going through real OIT. If you are considering being in a clinical trial you will have to accept this possibility and **if you can't accept being part of the placebo group then a clinical trial is not right for you.**

He came back and said, "To be considered for the trial you would have to change meds and come back for another round of skin tests." Now keep in mind this is a clinical research environment. This is not just their job it's their career. If I had lied about my anxiety or the medication I was using to treat it I would have been wasting their time and I'm sure they would have thanked me and shown me the door. But they didn't, they were giving me a second chance, and for that **I am truly grateful.**

Second try

I changed my meds as soon as I could and was stable on the new one for weeks before I had the chance to return for the repeat testing. This time was much better; the results were exactly as expected. I even announced on **Facebook,** "Hey, guess what? I just found out **I'm allergic to peanuts!**" Now I could schedule myself for the:

Double blind food challenge test

The procedure is simple. On two separate days they feed you either allergen or placebo and monitor your reaction. If you react you get treated, observed, and when it is CLINICALLY safe they let you leave. These are scheduled a week apart on the assumption that you will get an antihistamine on the first day and need a week to clear it from your system for the 2nd day.

Day 1

They put me on a bed. For the dosing I had to be on the bed. The little kid I was sharing the room with didn't have to be on the bed, she had toys and crayons and didn't have to be on a bed. I guess if she went ANA they could pick her up and treat her. Not so easy for an adult. But really, c'mon, no crayons??

I've got a blood ox monitor on my finger and a blood pressure cuff on my arm and they baseline me at 120/80. Really? 120/80? That's a little higher than I would expect, but ok. They keep checking in to see how I'm doing and they come back with the first dose in mixed in with applesauce. The protocol is dose, wait 15 min, then increase to the dose level. The first dose is 5mg, the second 20mg, and so on. "First a little on the lips, wait 30s, then lick your lips, wait again, then eat the dose." The procedure was amazingly similar to what I had already been doing the last 30 years. I'm sitting upright in the bed. She shows me the cup and label. It has my name on it. Then she reads the label to me:

"5mg of peanut protein."

I was actually going to eat peanuts. How surreal! I NEVER eat anything with a warning label that indicates even the slightest potential of cross contamination. First the lips.

"What do you feel?"

"Nothing" I replied.

Then I licked my lips. I tasted mostly applesauce and the oat flour. Then **there it was**, and *I thought the test would be over.*

"There's peanut in here, I can sense it."

"How do you know?"

"I feel it in my sinus"

"Anything else?"

"No"

"OK, **eat the rest**; I need to see a **visible** symptom"

Yikes! Exhale... I was afraid of this... not mentally afraid of actually eating the peanut, if that's what it really was, but I was afraid that my body/anxiety **wouldn't let me**. My years of preparing for this moment paid off, and I was able to swallow the rest of the mixture.

"So I thought this was supposed to be a double blind test, but I'm sure there is peanut in there"

"It doesn't matter what you believe, what's important is that I don't know which one it is. So, how are you feeling?"

I pause, I close my eyes, and I concentrate within to see if I can feel any reaction...

"Anxious"

"I know" said the doc, "**your blood pressure is 145,** just try to relax"

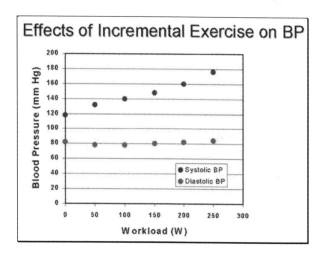

My body was responding as if I was taking a brisk jog, but I was sitting quietly in a hospital bed. Anxiety is a **silent killer** and if peanuts weren't going to kill me then anxiety surely would. **I needed this treatment.**

So I close my eyes and try to relax.

"But don't close your eyes and don't lie down"

Ok, I guess I have to meditate with my eyes open.

Tick, tick, tick ... The first dose is 5 milligrams; the next dose is four times bigger. Can I handle it? I really don't want to; please don't make me eat more peanut. One minute, two, three, four, and bingo, the lobster as cooked as a bright red rash appears on the back of my hands.

"OK, you are done, here, have some Zyrtec, we have to watch you for 2 more hours, then you can go."

And I was quite relieved that I didn't have to increase. I could relax and I felt tired. **Wow, this is not going to be easy**. I just hope this wasn't a psychosomatic reaction.

One week later

Same drill as before but I went in thinking "What if last week was PLACEBO? If that's the case then I'm out. Or what if since I believe that this is placebo that I don't react?" **Why do I have to over analyze everything??** I'm sitting upright in the bed. She shows me the cup and reads me the label

"5mg of peanut protein."

First the lips.

"What do you feel?"
"Nothing" I replied. Then I licked my lips. I tasted oats.
"What do you feel?"
"Anxious"
"Nothing else?"
"No"
"OK, eat the rest"

For the next four hours, every 15 minutes was a new dose which was mixed in applesauce. It was obvious the oat flavor was getting stronger as it progressed and my anxiety was gone. Even though before each dose she read the label and said I was eating peanut I knew it was not. I was relaxed and relieved. Then the dosing stopped and I still had to wait 2 more hours for observation. When everything was complete the study was un-blinded (converted to 'open label') and I had passed with flying colors. Now that the test was open label the doc was free to talk with me outside of the confines of the double blind test protocol, and she asked me a puzzling question. I later realized they work mostly with kids, so the question made more sense to me later. She asked:

"Since you reacted to peanut last time you knew this morning was placebo. Why were you anxious?"

I replied

"The label said it was peanuts. You read the label to me and told me I was eating peanuts"

And as she turned away I realized that

Allergists are not psychiatrists.

I was IN!

I was going for the last interview to be in the trial, speaking to a doctor who I hadn't talked with before. After that, sign the release for the OIT clinical study and schedule the first appointment. First, she described the goals of the research in detail, what they would be studying, how and why. An important 'arm' of this study was research on Eosinophilic Esophagitis (EoE) that involved endoscopic sampling through the course of the OIT trial, and as a matter of fact they had an opening the next day at the hospital for an endoscopy.

I checked my calendar and made that appointment on the spot. Be there 6:30, have someone to drive you home around nine am. I called my wife and made her cancel her morning clients.

We continued to talk a lot about anxiety and how that is one of their biggest concerns, because participants drop out over anxiety rather than physiological reasons. I explained in detail how I had that covered, it would not be a problem and I recounted the story when I was considering Phase 1 participation, but my anxiety wouldn't let me. The release form was pretty long, but pretty soon I got through it all and handed it off so they could make a copy for me.

I continued to talk about my avoidance protocols and how I never ate if I didn't have my epi-pen on me, and how in the last 30 years how I had left my epi at home at most twice, because going all day without eating sucks. She said, "Wow, you are the perfect patient." I also shared with her my experience being discharged from the ER after my 2nd reaction, something I have not yet written about, but intend to... someday. In reply she said,

> **"That probably saved your life. You know the population at greatest risk of fatal anaphylaxis is boys aged 18 to 25 because they think they are immortal."**

While waiting for the intern to bring back the forms we chatted about how the allergy had inhibited my life as an adult how I thought this would make such a difference for me. She looked up from what she was holding in her hand, stared me straight in the eye and with a look of excitement said,

> **"Well, I just want to tell you that OIT really, REALLY works!"**

I was ecstatic, I was overjoyed; I had HOPE for the first time in 30 years. This huge weight was lifted from my shoulders and I wasn't paying attention, but I heard myself say "no", "no", "no", "no", "no", but then I heard:

> *"FLUID REPLENISHMENT OR HYPOTENSION?"*

I hesitated, and looked to see she had been going down the list of exclusion criteria on the paper that she held in her hand. I said,

> "I don't remember ... it was a long time ago"

and we both knew I was lying.

In the brief moment before she turned away I saw a look of shock in her eyes, but I wasn't sure why.

Very delicately and with the kindest consideration for me an excuse was fabricated of why the endoscopy appointment was cancelled tomorrow, and they couldn't give me a firm answer on whether or not I could be part of the clinical trial, but they would check. This was March; I filled out the application the previous October and lied at the first interview in December. I hadn't read the trial requirements since then, and frankly, the change in my anxiety medication was taking some getting used to, mentally.

When I got home I dug up the document on the study, and the wording was unequivocal. There could be no exceptions to the exclusion criteria. This is when I came to the realization that when I was caught in the lie that I had dashed her hopes of helping me, because she knew she could, but wouldn't be allowed to. For that **I am truly sorry.**

I went to bed that night and woke up in the early morning as I had done so many times before, before getting fired and before anxiety treatment. When I woke up before I would be drenched in sweat, or have charlie horse cramps in one or both of my legs with heart pounding and gasping for air and I never knew why. But that early morning, about 2 am, March 20, 2015 I woke up with no physical symptoms. As I lay there it was all coming back to me, the reason why I lied and the reason why I had to lie, so I got out of bed, went to the keyboard and started typing and have continued to this day. The first words that appeared on the screen in front of me were:

I was sure I was going to die.

Glossary:

LTFA – Life Threatening Food Allergy

ANA – Anaphylactic

PN – Peanut

TN – Tree Nuts

IT – Immunotherapy
   – Desensitization by exposure to the allergen.
   Start small and slowly increase

OIT – Oral Immunotherapy – Allergen is eaten

SLIT – Sub Lingual
   – Allergen placed under the tongue

EPIT® - Epicutaneous IT
   – through the skin, a.k.a. the 'patch'
   - registered trademark of DVB Technologies

Resources:

Theories on LTFA

It would be impossible to list them all:

Peanut Allergy Epidemic -
> http://www.amazon.com/Peanut-Allergy-Epidemic-Whats-Causing/dp/1616082739/ref=sr_1_2

Food Babe Blog:
> http://thebitchywaiter.com/2014/07/this-woman-lies-about-allergies-and-is-fine-with-it.html

ADVANCED Acute management of anaphylaxis guidelines

These guidelines are intended for emergency department staff, ambulance staff, rural and remote GPs and nurses providing emergency care.

http://www.allergy.org.au/health-professionals/papers/advanced-acute-management-of-anaphylaxis-guidelines

Social Media:

The master list, grass roots support:
https://www.facebook.com/notes/peanut-anaphylaxis-cure/member-links-their-own-pages/586197604739256

Facebook Groups:

Peanut Anaphylaxis Cure
– One of the early/original groups

OIT 101 ← Start here for OIT

Private Practice OIT

OIT Trials

Peanut Allergy and Anaphylaxis Awareness
– Another early/original group

AFAxIT (LTFA & OIT, SLIT, EPIT)
- restricted to adults with LTFA

Airborne Anaphylaxis Is Real: A place for sharing stories...

Michiana Food Allergy & Anaphylaxis Chat Group

California State - Civil Rights for People with Anaphylaxis

Adult Food Allergic Support Group

SF Bay Area Food Allergy Network

Kids With Food Allergies Foundation

The International Men of Food Allergies

Non Profits:

FAACT - Food Allergy & Anaphylaxis Connection Team www.faact.com

FARE – Food Allergy Research and Education www.fare.org

AAFA – Asthma and Allergy Foundation of America www.aafa.org

Kids with Food Allergies, a subsidiary of AAFA

Get Schooled in Anaphylaxis: www.anaphylaxis101.com

Allergy Home - www.allergyhome.org

Anaphylaxis Canada: http://www.anaphylaxis.ca

Univ. of Nebraska FARRP – Food Allergy Research and Resource Program: https://farrp.unl.edu/informallbig8

False Prophets:

Peanut Allergy Facts – Funded by the National Peanut Board – A marketing organization for the peanut industry. They are disingenuous because they conveniently omit the fact that anaphylaxis can be fatal.

peanutallergyfacts.org

Airborne Exposure Research

This seems to be the original definitive work on the topic in 1999 and looks like not much more has been done since:

HTTP://WWW.NCBI.NLM.NIH.GOV/PUBMED/10400859

SELF-REPORTED ALLERGIC REACTIONS TO PEANUT ON COMMERCIAL AIRLINERS.

Authors: **Sicherer SH**[1]**, Furlong TJ, DeSimone J, Sampson HA**.

BACKGROUND:
Allergic reactions to food occurring on commercial airlines have not been systematically characterized.

OBJECTIVE:
We sought to describe the clinical characteristics of allergic reactions to peanuts on airplanes.

METHODS:
Participants in the National Registry of Peanut and Tree Nut Allergy who indicated an allergic reaction while on a commercial airliner were interviewed by telephone.

RESULTS:
Sixty-two of 3704 National Registry of Peanut and Tree Nut Allergy participants indicated a reaction on an airplane; 42 of 48 patients or parental surrogates contacted confirmed the reaction began on the airplane (median age of affected subject, 2 years;

range, 6 months to 50 years). Of these, 35 reacted to peanuts (4 were uncertain of exposure) and 7 to tree nuts, although 3 of these 7 reacted to substances that may have also contained peanut. Exposures occurred by ingestion (20 subjects), skin contact (8 subjects), and inhalation (14 subjects). Reactions generally occurred within 10 minutes of exposure (32 of 42 subjects), and reaction severity correlated with exposure route (ingestion > inhalation > skin). The causal food was generally served by the airline (37 of 42 subjects). Medications were given in flight to 19 patients (epinephrine to 5) and to an additional 14 at landing/gate return (including epinephrine to 1 and intravenous medication to 2), totaling 79% treated. Flight crews were notified in 33% of reactions. During inhalation reactions as a result of peanut allergy, greater than 25 passengers were estimated to be eating peanuts at the time of the reaction. Initial symptoms generally involved the upper airway, with progression to the skin or further lower respiratory reactions (no gastrointestinal symptoms).

CONCLUSIONS:

Allergic reactions to peanuts and tree nuts caused by accidental ingestion, skin contact, or inhalation occur during commercial flights, but airline personnel are usually not notified. Reactions can be severe, requiring medications, including epinephrine.

Airline snack foods: tension in the peanut gallery. [J Allergy Clin Immunol. 1999]

PMID: 10400859 [PubMed - indexed for MEDLINE]

Good Doggy Kisses

"We essentially want to find out, is a dog acting like yogurt in having a probiotic effect?" Kim Kelly, an anthropology doctoral student involved in the study told **The Independent**.

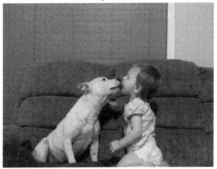

"We think dogs might work as probiotics to enhance the health of the bacteria that live in our guts. These bacteria, or 'microbiota,' are increasingly recognized as playing an essential role in our mental and physical health, especially as we age," said Dr. Charles Raison, principal investigator for the study and a UA professor of psychiatry in the College of Medicine.

Other studies have shown that dogs and their owners share much of the same gut bacteria over time, which **helps people ward off allergies**. Another study by Finnish scientists **found that babies in homes with dogs** were found to have fewer colds, fewer ear infections, and need fewer antibiotics in their first year of life than babies raised in pet-free homes.

Read more at :
> http://www.dogheirs.com/dogheirs/posts/662
> 5-dog-kisses-may-improve-your-health
>
> http://www.youtube.com/watch?v=O1oHfR
> dtgwk

See how an Epi-pen is constructed:
> http://cdn1.m3design.com/wordpress/wp-
> content/uploads/2014/03/Product-Teardown-
> EpiPen-v3.pdf

Auto-injector racketeering:
> http://inthesetimes.com/article/16951/anaphy
> lactic_sticker_shock

Epilogue

I have learned so much in such a short time. Thank you for letting me share my story.

Michael

19846859R00069